I0090157

Environmental Health Criteria 22_

NEUROTOXICITY RISK ASSESSMENT FOR HUMAN HEALTH: PRINCIPLES AND APPROACHES

First draft prepared by Dr J. Harry, US National Institute of Environmental Health Sciences, Research Triangle Park, North Carolina, USA; Dr B. Kulig, Kulig Consultancy, The Netherlands; Dr M. Lotti, University of Padua, Italy; Dr D. Ray, MRC Toxicology Unit, England; Dr H. Tilson, US Environmental Protection Agency, Research Triangle Park, North Carolina, USA; and Dr G. Winneke, Medical Institute of Environmental Hygiene, Germany

Published under the joint sponsorship of the United Nations Environment Programme, the International Labour Organization and the World Health Organization, and produced within the framework of the Inter-Organization Programme for the Sound Management of Chemicals.

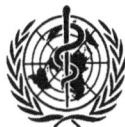

World Health Organization
Geneva, 2001

The **International Programme on Chemical Safety (IPCS)**, established in 1980, is a joint venture of the United Nations Environment Programme (UNEP), the International Labour Organization (ILO) and the World Health Organization (WHO). The overall objectives of the IPCS are to establish the scientific basis for assessment of the risk to human health and the environment from exposure to chemicals, through international peer review processes, as a prerequisite for the promotion of chemical safety, and to provide technical assistance in strengthening national capacities for the sound management of chemicals.

The **Inter-Organization Programme for the Sound Management of Chemicals (IOMC)** was established in 1995 by UNEP, ILO, the Food and Agriculture Organization of the United Nations, WHO, the United Nations Industrial Development Organization, the United Nations Institute for Training and Research and the Organisation for Economic Co-operation and Development (Participating Organizations), following recommendations made by the 1992 UN Conference on Environment and Development to strengthen cooperation and increase coordination in the field of chemical safety. The purpose of the IOMC is to promote coordination of the policies and activities pursued by the Participating Organizations, jointly or separately, to achieve the sound management of chemicals in relation to human health and the environment.

WHO Library Cataloguing-in-Publication Data

Neurotoxicity risk assessment for human health : principles and approaches.

(Environmental health criteria ; 223)

1.Nervous system - drug effects 2.Chemicals - toxicity 3.Neurotoxicity syndromes - etiology 4.Risk assessment - methods 5.Environmental exposure I.International Programme for Chemical Safety II.Series

ISBN 92 4 157223 X   (NLM classification: WL 100)
ISSN 0250-863X

The World Health Organization welcomes requests for permission to reproduce or translate its publications, in part or in full. Applications and enquiries should be addressed to the Office of Publications, World Health Organization, Geneva, Switzerland, which will be glad to provide the latest information on any changes made to the text, plans for new editions, and reprints and translations already available.

Printed in Finland
2001/13704 – Vammala – 5000

CONTENTS

**ENVIRONMENTAL HEALTH CRITERIA FOR
NEUROTOXICITY RISK ASSESSMENT FOR HUMAN
HEALTH: PRINCIPLES AND APPROACHES**

NOTE TO READERS OF THE CRITERIA MONOGRAPHS

Every effort has been made to present information in the criteria monographs as accurately as possible without unduly delaying their publication. In the interest of all users of the Environmental Health Criteria monographs, readers are requested to communicate any errors that may have occurred to the Director of the International Programme on Chemical Safety, World Health Organization, Geneva, Switzerland, in order that they may be included in corrigenda.

* * *

A detailed data profile and a legal file can be obtained from the International Register of Potentially Toxic Chemicals, Case postale 356, 1219 Châtelaine, Geneva, Switzerland (telephone no. + 41 22 – 9799111, fax no. + 41 22 – 7973460, E-mail irptc@unep.ch).

Environmental Health Criteria

PREAMBLE

Objectives

In 1973, the WHO Environmental Health Criteria Programme was initiated with the following objectives:

(i)   to assess information on the relationship between exposure to environmental pollutants and human health, and to provide guidelines for setting exposure limits;

(ii) to identify new or potential pollutants;

(iii) to identify gaps in knowledge concerning the health effects of pollutants;

(iv) to promote the harmonization of toxicological and epidemiological methods in order to have internationally comparable results.

The first Environmental Health Criteria (EHC) monograph, on mercury, was published in 1976, and since that time an ever-increasing number of assessments of chemicals and of physical effects have been produced. In addition, many EHC monographs have been devoted to evaluating toxicological methodology, e.g., for genetic, neurotoxic, teratogenic and nephrotoxic effects. Other publications have been concerned with epidemiological guidelines, evaluation of short-term tests for carcinogens, biomarkers, effects on the elderly and so forth.

Since its inauguration, the EHC Programme has widened its scope, and the importance of environmental effects, in addition to health effects, has been increasingly emphasized in the total evaluation of chemicals.

The original impetus for the Programme came from World Health Assembly resolutions and the recommendations of the 1972 UN Conference on the Human Environment. Subsequently, the work became an integral part of the International Programme on Chemical

Safety (IPCS), a cooperative programme of UNEP, ILO and WHO. In this manner, with the strong support of the new partners, the importance of occupational health and environmental effects was fully recognized. The EHC monographs have become widely established, used and recognized throughout the world.

The recommendations of the 1992 UN Conference on Environment and Development and the subsequent establishment of the Intergovernmental Forum on Chemical Safety with the priorities for action in the six programme areas of Chapter 19, Agenda 21, all lend further weight to the need for EHC assessments of the risks of chemicals.

Scope

The criteria monographs are intended to provide critical reviews on the effects on human health and the environment of chemicals and of combinations of chemicals and physical and biological agents. As such, they include and review studies that are of direct relevance for the evaluation. However, they do not describe *every* study carried out. Worldwide data are used and are quoted from original studies, not from abstracts or reviews. Both published and unpublished reports are considered, and it is incumbent on the authors to assess all the articles cited in the references. Preference is always given to published data. Unpublished data are used only when relevant published data are absent or when they are pivotal to the risk assessment. A detailed policy statement is available that describes the procedures used for unpublished proprietary data so that this information can be used in the evaluation without compromising its confidential nature (WHO (1990) Revised Guidelines for the Preparation of Environmental Health Criteria Monographs. PCS/90.69, Geneva, World Health Organization).

In the evaluation of human health risks, sound human data, whenever available, are preferred to animal data. Animal and *in vitro* studies provide support and are used mainly to supply evidence missing from human studies. It is mandatory that research on human subjects is conducted in full accord with ethical principles, including the provisions of the Helsinki Declaration.

The EHC monographs are intended to assist national and international authorities in making risk assessments and subsequent risk management decisions. They represent a thorough evaluation of risks and are not, in any sense, recommendations for regulation or standard setting. These latter are the exclusive purview of national and regional governments.

Content

The layout of EHC monographs for chemicals is outlined below.

- Summary — a review of the salient facts and the risk evaluation of the chemical
- Identity — physical and chemical properties, analytical methods
- Sources of exposure
- Environmental transport, distribution and transformation
- Environmental levels and human exposure
- Kinetics and metabolism in laboratory animals and humans
- Effects on laboratory mammals and *in vitro* test systems
- Effects on humans
- Effects on other organisms in the laboratory and field
- Evaluation of human health risks and effects on the environment
- Conclusions and recommendations for protection of human health and the environment
- Further research
- Previous evaluations by international bodies, e.g., IARC, JECFA, JMPR

Selection of chemicals

Since the inception of the EHC Programme, the IPCS has organized meetings of scientists to establish lists of priority chemicals for subsequent evaluation. Such meetings have been held in: Ispra, Italy, 1980; Oxford, United Kingdom, 1984; Berlin, Germany, 1987; and North Carolina, USA, 1995. The selection of chemicals has been based on the following criteria: the existence of scientific evidence that the substance presents a hazard to human health and/or the environment; the possible use, persistence, accumulation or degradation of the substance shows that there may be significant human or environmental exposure; the size and nature of populations at risk (both human and other species) and risks for the environment; international concern, i.e., the substance is of major interest to several countries; adequate data on the hazards are available.

If an EHC monograph is proposed for a chemical not on the priority list, the IPCS Secretariat consults with the cooperating organizations and all the Participating Institutions before embarking on the preparation of the monograph.

Procedures

The order of procedures that result in the publication of an EHC monograph is shown in the flow chart. A designated staff member of IPCS, responsible for the scientific quality of the document, serves as Responsible Officer (RO). The IPCS Editor is responsible for layout and language. The first draft, prepared by consultants or, more usually, staff from an IPCS Participating Institution, is based initially on data provided from the International Register of Potentially Toxic Chemicals and from reference databases such as Medline and Toxline.

The draft document, when received by the RO, may require an initial review by a small panel of experts to determine its scientific quality and objectivity. Once the RO finds the document acceptable as a first draft, it is distributed, in its unedited form, to well over 150 EHC contact points throughout the world who are asked to comment on its completeness and accuracy and, where necessary, provide additional material. The contact points, usually designated by governments, may be Participating Institutions, IPCS Focal Points or individual scientists known for their particular expertise. Generally, some four months are allowed before the comments are considered by the RO and author(s). A second draft incorporating comments received and approved by the Director, IPCS, is then distributed to Task Group members, who carry out the peer review, at least six weeks before their meeting.

The Task Group members serve as individual scientists, not as representatives of any organization, government or industry. Their function is to evaluate the accuracy, significance and relevance of the

EHC PREPARATION FLOW CHART

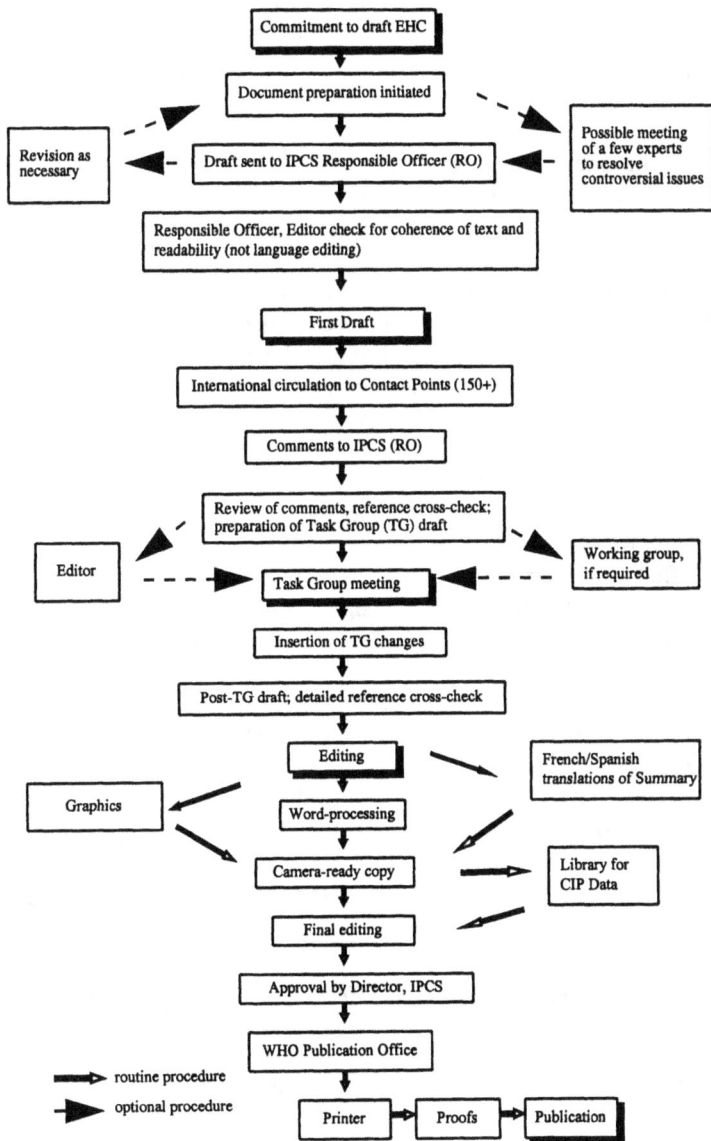

```
                    ┌─────────────────────────┐
                    │  Commitment to draft EHC │
                    └─────────────────────────┘
                                 │
                    ┌─────────────────────────┐
                    │ Document preparation initiated │
                    └─────────────────────────┘
```

Commitment to draft EHC

Document preparation initiated

Revision as necessary

Draft sent to IPCS Responsible Officer (RO)

Possible meeting of a few experts to resolve controversial issues

Responsible Officer, Editor check for coherence of text and readability (not language editing)

First Draft

International circulation to Contact Points (150+)

Comments to IPCS (RO)

Review of comments, reference cross-check; preparation of Task Group (TG) draft

Editor

Working group, if required

Task Group meeting

Insertion of TG changes

Post-TG draft; detailed reference cross-check

Editing

French/Spanish translations of Summary

Graphics

Word-processing

Camera-ready copy

Library for CIP Data

Final editing

Approval by Director, IPCS

WHO Publication Office

routine procedure

optional procedure

Printer

Proofs

Publication

information in the document and to assess the health and environmental risks from exposure to the chemical. A summary and recommendations for further research and improved safety aspects are also required. The composition of the Task Group is dictated by the range of expertise required for the subject of the meeting and by the need for a balanced geographical distribution.

The three cooperating organizations of the IPCS recognize the important role played by nongovernmental organizations. Representatives from relevant national and international associations may be invited to join the Task Group as observers. While observers may provide a valuable contribution to the process, they can speak only at the invitation of the Chairperson. Observers do not participate in the final evaluation of the chemical; this is the sole responsibility of the Task Group members. When the Task Group considers it to be appropriate, it may meet *in camera*.

All individuals who as authors, consultants or advisers participate in the preparation of the EHC monograph must, in addition to serving in their personal capacity as scientists, inform the RO if at any time a conflict of interest, whether actual or potential, could be perceived in their work. They are required to sign a conflict of interest statement. Such a procedure ensures the transparency and probity of the process.

When the Task Group has completed its review and the RO is satisfied as to the scientific correctness and completeness of the document, the document then goes for language editing, reference checking and preparation of camera-ready copy. After approval by the Director, IPCS, the monograph is submitted to the WHO Office of Publications for printing. At this time, a copy of the final draft is sent to the Chairperson and Rapporteur of the Task Group to check for any errors.

It is accepted that the following criteria should initiate the updating of an EHC monograph: new data are available that would substantially change the evaluation; there is public concern for health or environmental effects of the agent because of greater exposure; an appreciable time period has elapsed since the last evaluation.

All Participating Institutions are informed, through the EHC progress report, of the authors and institutions proposed for the drafting of the documents. A comprehensive file of all comments received on drafts of each EHC monograph is maintained and is available on request. The Chairpersons of Task Groups are briefed before each meeting on their role and responsibility in ensuring that these rules are followed.

WHO TASK GROUP ON ENVIRONMENTAL HEALTH CRITERIA FOR NEUROTOXICITY RISK ASSESSMENT FOR HUMAN HEALTH: PRINCIPLES AND APPROACHES

Members

Dr S.A. Assimon, US Food and Drug Administration, USA

Dr R. Duffard, Laboratorio de Toxicologia Experimental, Argentina

Dr J. Harry, US National Institute of Environmental Health Sciences, USA

Dr B. Kulig, Kulig Consultancy, The Netherlands

Dr O. Ladefoged, Institute of Food Safety and Toxicology, Denmark

Dr M. Lotti, University of Padova, Italy

Dr J. O'Donoghue, Eastman Kodak Company, USA

Dr D. Ray, MRC Toxicology Unit, United Kingdom

Dr J. Ross, Procter & Gamble Company (representing American Industrial Health Council)

Dr H. Tilson, US Environmental Protection Agency, USA *(Chair)*

Dr G. Winneke, Medical Institute of Environmental Hygiene, Germany

Secretariat

Dr T. Damstra, World Health Organization, IPCS/Interregional Research Unit (IRRU), USA

PREFACE

The IPCS, initiated in 1980 as a collaborative programme of UNEP, the ILO, and WHO, has as one of its major objectives the development and evaluation of principles and methodologies for assessing the effects of chemicals on human health and the environment. Since its inception, IPCS has given high priority to improving scientific methodologies and promoting internationally accepted strategies to assess the risks from exposure to neurotoxic chemicals.

In 1986, IPCS published the EHC document entitled "Principles and Methods for the Assessment of Neurotoxicity Associated with Exposure to Chemicals" (IPCS, 1986). This publication focused on neurobehavioural, neurophysiological, neurochemical and neuropathological methods that had been successfully applied in neurotoxicity studies. The recommendations contained in the 1986 EHC led to a WHO/IPCS-sponsored multilaboratory, collaborative study to ascertain whether a standardized neurobehavioural examination could be developed to assess the effects of chemicals. Several established endpoints for neurotoxicity and some well known neurotoxicants were selected in order to assess the validity both within and across laboratories in detecting the neurobehavioural effects (MacPhail et al., 1997). The results of this collaborative study strongly supported the use of behavioural tests for the screening of neurotoxicity and were incorporated into the Neurotoxicity Risk Assessment Guidelines of the US Environmental Protection Agency (EPA) and the Organisation for Economic Co-operation and Development (OECD) Test Guidelines for neurotoxicity testing.

Since 1986, new advances in basic neurobiology research and in the development of new technologies have significantly improved our ability to assess the neurotoxic potential of chemicals. The availability of up-to-date principles and approaches on neurotoxicity is the subject of urgent requests from many countries, and IPCS was advised to update the 1986 publication.

This document addresses the major scientific principles underlying hazard identification, testing methods and risk assessment strategies in assessing human neurotoxicity. It provides an overview of the current state of neurotoxicity risk assessment for public health officials, research and regulatory scientists, and risk managers. It is intended to complement existing monographs, reviews and test guidelines (OECD, 1995, 1997, 1999; Sobotka et al., 1996; Babich, 1998; US EPA, 1998a). It is not intended to be prescriptive in nature or a textbook on neurotoxicology.

A preliminary draft of the document was circulated to 64 experts in neurotoxicology and IPCS contact points for their review. Many reviewers provided substantive comments and text, and their contributions are gratefully acknowledged.

A Task Group meeting was held in Washington, DC, on 29–31 March 2000, to review a revised draft. Dr Damstra, IPCS, was responsible for the preparation of the final document and for its overall scientific content.

The efforts of all who helped in the preparation and finalization of the monograph are gratefully acknowledged. Special thanks are due to the US EPA and the US National Institute of Environmental Health Sciences for their financial support for the planning and review group meetings.

ACRONYMS AND ABBREVIATIONS

AChE	acetylcholinesterase
ADI	acceptable daily intake
AENTB	Adult Environmental Neurobehavioral Test Battery
ALS	amyotrophic lateral sclerosis
ATP	adenosine triphosphate
ATPase	adenosine triphosphatase
BAEP	brainstem auditory evoked potential
BBB	blood–brain barrier
BMD	benchmark dose
CAT	computerized axial tomography
CNS	central nervous system
CPA	cyclopiazonic acid
CSEP	chemosensory evoked potential
CSF	cerebrospinal fluid
CVO	circumventricular organ
DNA	deoxyribonucleic acid
EAA	excitatory amino acid
EC	European Commission
ECETOC	European Centre for Ecotoxicology and Toxicology of Chemicals
EEG	electroencephalography/electroencephalograph
EHC	Environmental Health Criteria
EMG	electromyography/electromyograph
EP	evoked potential
EPA	Environmental Protection Agency (USA)
ERP	event-related potential
EU	European Union
FAO	Food and Agriculture Organization of the United Nations
FDA	Food and Drug Administration (USA)
FOB	functional observational battery
GABA	γ-aminobutyric acid
GCP	Good Clinical Practice
GFAP	glial fibrillary acidic protein
HSP	heat shock protein
IARC	International Agency for Research on Cancer
ILO	International Labour Organization

IPCS	International Programme on Chemical Safety
IQ	intelligence quotient
JECFA	Joint FAO/WHO Expert Committee on Food Additives
JEM	job exposure matrix
JMPR	Joint FAO/WHO Meeting on Pesticide Residues
LOAEL	lowest-observed-adverse-effect level
LTP	long-term potentiation
MCV	motor conduction velocity
MMPI-R	Minnesota Multiphasic Personality Inventory (revised)
MOE	margin of exposure
MPTP	1-methyl-4-phenyl-1,2,3,6-tetrahydropyridine
MRI	magnetic resonance imaging
mRNA	messenger ribonucleic acid
NAP	nerve action potential
NCTB	Neurobehavioural Core Test Battery
NCV	nerve conduction velocity
NES	Neurobehavioural Evaluation System
NOAEL	no-observed-adverse-effect level
NRC	National Research Council (USA)
NSC-60	Neurotoxic Symptom Checklist-60
NTE	neuropathy target enzyme
OECD	Organisation for Economic Co-operation and Development
OPIDN	organophosphate-induced delayed neuropathy
PBB	polybrominated biphenyl
PBPK	physiologically based pharmacokinetic
PCB	polychlorinated biphenyl
PET	positron emission tomography
PNS	peripheral nervous system
POMS	Profile of Mood States
qEEG	quantitative electroencephalography
RfC	reference concentration
RfD	reference dose
RO	Responsible Officer
SAR	structure–activity relationship
SCOB	schedule-controlled operant behaviour
SEP	sensory evoked potential
SHE	sentinel health event

SPECT	single photon emission computerized tomography
SPES	Swedish Performance Evaluation System
SSEP	somatosensory evoked potential
TDI	tolerable daily intake
TOCP	tri-*o*-cresylphosphate
UN	United Nations
UNEP	United Nations Environment Programme
VEP	visual evoked potential
WAIS-R	Wechsler Adult Intelligence Scale (revised)
WHO	World Health Organization

1. SUMMARY AND RECOMMENDATIONS

1.1 Summary

Since the 1986 publication of the IPCS Environmental Health Criteria document on "Principles and Methods for the Assessment of Neurotoxicity Associated with Exposure to Chemicals," basic research in neurobiology has significantly improved our ability to assess how chemicals may adversely affect the nervous system. This progress is reflected in the availability of a number of national and international (e.g., Organisation for Economic Co-operation and Development) neurotoxicity test guidelines, risk assessment guidelines and guidance documents and international neurobehavioural test method validation studies.

Even with the improvements made in neurotoxicity risk assessment, there is still worldwide concern about the potential neurotoxic effects of chemicals. Of particular concern is the lack of data on putative relationships between exposures to low levels of environmental chemicals and effects on neurobehavioural development in children and neurodegenerative diseases in the elderly. Only a small fraction of chemicals have been adequately evaluated for neurotoxicity.

The complexity of the nervous system results in multiple potential target sites and adverse sequelae. No other organ system has the wide variety of specialized cell functions seen in the nervous system. Different expressions of neurotoxicity are generally based on the different susceptibilities of the various subpopulations of cells that make up the nervous system. The status and role of the blood–brain barrier in the central nervous system (CNS) and similar structures in the peripheral nervous system in modulating the access of some chemicals to the nervous system are also unique considerations in assessing neurotoxicity. Moreover, certain specialized cells outside the barrier have important integrative neuro-immuno-endocrine functions that orchestrate numerous physiological, metabolic and endocrine processes. These integrative functions are fundamental for cognition and higher-order neural functions, but knowledge on how they can be disrupted by chemical exposures is limited. In contrast to other tissues, the ability of nerve cells to replace or regenerate is severely constrained and is a limiting factor in achieving full recovery from neurotoxicity under conditions where cell death has occurred.

The biological basis for identification of certain susceptible populations, including the young, the aged and people with genetic predispositions to certain forms of toxicity, is an important consideration in the risk assessment process for neurotoxicity. Many of the factors that convey susceptibility for neurotoxicity will not differ from those that need to be considered in risk assessments of toxicity to other target organs, because they involve metabolic processes that are common to many organ systems. However, the complexity and critically timed events of the long postnatal CNS development process may make the developing nervous system differentially susceptible to certain exposures. Also, the aging process results in a reduction of plasticity and diminished compensatory capacity of the nervous system, making it potentially more susceptible to neurotoxic insults.

Data on the effects of chemicals on humans are often not available or are underreported. The detection of neurotoxicity in human studies provides the most direct means of assessing health risk, but is often complicated by confounding factors and inadequate data. Exposure levels in humans are difficult to establish, and the neurological status of populations is extremely heterogeneous. Nevertheless, there has been significant progress in the last decade in developing validated methods for detecting neurotoxicity in humans. Sources of human data include accidental and occupational exposures, case-studies, clinical evaluations, epidemiological studies, and field and laboratory studies. Standardized neuropsychological tests, validated computer-assisted test batteries, neurophysiological and biochemical tests, and refined imaging techniques have been improved and become well established. These methods can be used to assess a variety of human neurotoxic end-points and have provided useful data for the purpose of neurotoxicity risk assessment.

For most neurotoxicological assessments, it is still necessary to rely on information derived from experimental animal models. Behavioural, biochemical, electrophysiological and histopathological methods, along with validated batteries of functional tests, are now routinely used in animal studies to identify and characterize neurotoxic effects. Standardization and validation of animal test batteries have improved the quality of the data available for risk assessment. Using various combinations of these methods, specific testing protocols, test guidelines and testing strategies for neurotoxicity in adults and developing animals have been developed by intergovernmental organizations and national governments. New guidelines for standard acute and repeated-dose toxicity studies now also include behavioural and histopathological end-points specifically intended to improve the evaluation of the nervous system. Although animal models have been used extensively to study the differential sensitivity of developing organisms to chemical insults, current guidelines for developmental neurotoxicity are complex, and the results are often subject to varying interpretations. Most neurotoxicity testing strategies use a hierarchical or tiered approach. However, in addition to test protocol data, all available sources of data (structure–activity relationships, mechanistic research, etc.) must be considered to provide in-depth information about a specific type of neurotoxic effect.

As with other toxicities, a variety of factors are critical considerations in evaluating the neurotoxic potential of chemicals in experimental animals. These include selection of the appropriate animal models, exposure variables and test methods, an understanding of the biological relevance of the end-points being measured, use of validated measures and quality assurance. The experimental conditions should take into account the potential route and level of human exposure and any available information on toxicodynamics and toxicokinetics.

Many countries have developed risk assessment processes in which relevant data on the biological effects, dose–response relationships and exposure for a particular chemical are analysed in an attempt to establish qualitative and quantitative estimates of adverse outcomes. These processes are relatively similar and typically include hazard identification, dose–response evaluation, exposure assessment and risk characterization. Although principles of risk assessment specifically for neurotoxicity are evolving rapidly, they are still generally limited to qualitative hazard identification and, to some extent, dose–response assessment. Only a few assessments adequately cover exposure assessment or risk characterization.

The application of risk assessment principles for neurotoxic chemicals is generally similar to that for other non-cancer end-points except that issues of reversibility, compensation and redundancy of function in the nervous system require special consideration. Conventionally, neurotoxicological risk assessments have been based on no-observed-adverse-effect levels and empirical uncertainty factors to derive acceptable exposure limits. The evaluation of all available data is the key to providing sound risk assessments. Test methods and strategies in animals need to be continually refined as new data and technologies become available so as to improve the predictive validity of animal models for human neurotoxicity risk assessment.

1.2 Recommendations

In order to employ effective control and intervention strategies to prevent human neurotoxicity, an adequate knowledge base on potential neurotoxicity of chemicals must be developed. The following recommendations are made to improve this knowledge base:

1. Surveillance programmes and the use of harmonized formats for the collection of data on the incidence of poisonings and adverse reactions to neurotoxic agents in humans should be promoted and strengthened.

2. Better assessment of exposure of individuals and of populations to neurotoxic agents is needed in order to analyse associations between exposure and effect.

3. There is a need to conduct hypothesis-based epidemiological and experimental studies on the potential association between environmental exposures and neurodegenerative diseases, particularly as it relates to susceptible populations and gene–environment interactions.

4. Biomarkers of exposure, effect and susceptibility should be identified, developed and validated for use in epidemiological studies of neurotoxicity.

5. Research efforts are needed to better identify subpopulations that are potentially susceptible to the effects of neurotoxic agents and to characterize the factors contributing to increased susceptibility.

6. Standardized test methods and the development of norms for evaluating neurotoxicity in infants and children are needed for use in cross-cultural studies of human developmental neurotoxicity.

7. More emphasis should be placed on studies involving perinatal exposure to chemicals and/or mixtures of chemicals to define the relative sensitivity of the developing nervous system to neurotoxic injury.

8. Efficient animal testing approaches for developmental neurotoxicity need to be developed and validated in international collaborative studies.

9. In order to establish the biological significance of the subtle changes in many of the end-points used in neurotoxicology research efforts, improved animal models are needed to elucidate the relationships between molecular/cellular events and the clinical manifestations of neurotoxicity.

10. Research on how chemicals affect the integrated functions of the nervous system, particularly research related to endocrine disruptors, should be promoted.

11. There is a need for further exploration of the value of utilizing structure–activity relationships in identifying the neurotoxic potential of chemicals.

12. In order to reduce the uncertainties in current neurotoxicity risk assessment associated with the reliance on default assumptions and uncertainty factors for extrapolating from animal to human and from acute to chronic, as well as to account for variability within populations, research is needed to (1) delineate mechanisms of neurotoxicity and promote the use of mechanistic data in assessing risk; (2) provide mechanistically based dose–response models and toxicokinetic models that allow for extrapolation across dose, route and species; (3) reduce the use of uncertainty factors in quantitative risk assessment calculations; and (4) promote the availability and use of improved and harmonized risk assessment procedures.

5

13. Current risk assessment guidelines focus on assessing single chemicals following exposure via single pathways. In order to address aggregate exposure or cumulative toxicity issues, research is needed to (1) test the hypothesis of additivity for chemicals having a similar mode of action; (2) assess possible non-additive interactions of chemicals with different modes of action; and (3) study potential interactions of multiple chemicals at doses below those required to produce detectable effects following single exposures.

2. INTRODUCTION

Chemicals have become an indispensable part of human life, sustaining activities and development, preventing and controlling many diseases, and increasing agricultural productivity. Despite their benefits, chemicals may, especially when misused, cause adverse effects on human health. The nervous system has been shown to be particularly vulnerable to certain chemical exposures, and there is increasing global concern about the potential health effects from exposure to neurotoxic chemicals.

There is a lack of available toxicological data for many compounds used commercially, and most chemicals have not been adequately assessed for their neurotoxic potential (US NRC, 1984). The need for a multidisciplinary approach to neurotoxicity risk assessment has been recognized by a number of international and scientific organizations and national governments (IPCS, 1986b; Landrigan et al., 1994; OECD, 1995, 1997, 1999; Simonsen et al., 1995; LeBel & Foss, 1996; SGOMSEC, 1996; Sobotka et al., 1996; Chouaniere et al., 1997; US EPA, 1998a).

2.1 Purpose of the publication

This publication summarizes the scientific knowledge base on which principles and methods involved in neurotoxicity risk assessment are based. It is aimed at providing a framework for public health officials, research and regulatory scientists, and risk managers on the use and interpretation of neurotoxicity data from human and animal studies, and it discusses emerging methodological approaches to studying neurotoxicity. It does not provide practical advice or specific guidance for the conduct of specific tests and studies. These guidelines have been developed and issued by international organizations and national governments and vary depending on the types of chemicals being assessed and on national regulations and recommendations.

The Organisation for Economic Co-operation and Development (OECD) has developed internationally agreed-upon Test Guidelines for the testing of chemicals for potential neurotoxicity. OECD is an intergovernmental organization of 29 industrialized countries in North

America, Europe and the Pacific, as well as the European Commission (EC), which meet to coordinate and harmonize policies and work together to respond to international concerns. Specific OECD Test Guidelines include those for single-dose toxicity (e.g., OECD 402, 403, 420 and 423) (OECD, 1981, 1987a, 1992, 1996) and repeated-dose toxicity (e.g., OECD 405 and 408) (OECD, 1987b, 1998), as well as Test Guidelines specifically developed for the study of neurotoxicity in adult and young laboratory animals (i.e., OECD 418, 419, 424 and 426) (OECD, 1995, 1997, 1999). OECD is also developing a Guidance Document on Neurotoxicity Testing (in preparation) to ensure that sufficient data are obtained to enable adequate evaluation of the risks of neurotoxicity. The European Union (EC, 1996), European Centre for Ecotoxicology and Toxicology of Chemicals (ECETOC, 1992), US Food and Drug Administration (US FDA, 1970), US Environmental Protection Agency (US EPA, 1998a) and US Consumer Product Safety Commission (Babich, 1998) have also developed testing strategy and evaluation guidelines. In addition, the Danish Environmental Protection Agency (Ladefoged et al., 1995) issued a document on criteria for evaluating neurotoxicity.

This document does not elaborate in detail on developmental neurotoxicology, since issues related to this topic are being addressed in the revised OECD Test Guideline 426: Developmental Neurotoxicity Study (OECD, 1999) and in another IPCS publication, "Principles for Evaluating Human Reproductive Effects of Chemicals" (in preparation). It also does not address in detail recent research and international concerns about the potential adverse developmental and neurotoxic effects from exposure to chemicals that have the potential to disrupt the endocrine system (Kavlock et al., 1996; IUPAC, 1998; EC, 1999; US NRC, 1999). Data on endocrine disrupting chemicals are currently being evaluated in another IPCS monograph, "Global Assessment of the State-of-the-Science of Endocrine Disruptors" (in preparation).

This document also reviews methods for evaluating effects and deriving exposure guidelines when neurotoxicity is a critical effect. The availability of alternative mathematical approaches to dose–response analyses, characterization of the health-related database for neurotoxicity risk assessment, and the integration of exposure information with results of the dose–response assessment to characterize risks are also discussed.

The present chapter provides an overview of the magnitude of the problem, defines key terms and discusses critical concepts, assumptions and criteria for neurotoxicity risk assessment. Chapter 3 discusses basic principles of neurobiology and toxicology that could be useful for risk assessors seeking to understand the scientific basis for specific methods and procedures used in neurotoxicology and the relative vulnerability of specific structures and processes that are essential for normal functioning of the nervous system. This chapter also provides basic toxicological principles concerning how chemicals can interact with the nervous system. In addition, Chapter 3 describes the potential for subpopulations within the larger population to be differentially sensitive to chemical exposure and ends with a general overview of the various types of adverse effects that chemicals can have on the structure and function of the nervous system. Chapter 4 covers an area of neurotoxicology that was not addressed in the 1986 IPCS document: human neurotoxicology. This chapter describes the general procedures that are commonly used to assess chemical effects in humans and discusses important issues of experimental design and data interpretation. Chapter 5 describes the interpretation of data from animal studies. Methods used to assess neurotoxicity in animals were covered in great detail in the 1986 IPCS document, while the present document focuses more on guidance concerning the interpretation of results from such methods. This chapter also includes examples of chemicals that at some dose are known to affect behavioural, neurochemical, neurophysiological or neuroanatomical end-points in animal models. Chapter 6 deals with the emerging area of neurotoxicity risk assessment. This chapter discusses the four-step risk assessment process described by the US National Research Council (US NRC, 1983) and is intended to provide principles that can be used to assess in a qualitative and quantitative manner human health risk based on data from human and animal studies.

2.2 General principles of neurotoxicity risk assessment

Risk assessment is a process intended to identify and then to calculate or estimate the risk for a given target system to be affected by a particular substance, taking into account the inherent characteristics of the substance of concern as well as the characteristics of the specific target system. Risk management is a decision-making process involving considerations of political, social, economic and technical factors with relevant risk assessment information relating to a hazard so as to develop, analyse and compare regulatory and non-regulatory options and to select and implement the optimal response for safety from that hazard. Hazard refers to the inherent property of a substance capable of having adverse effects (OECD/IPCS, 2001).

Neurotoxicity is one of several non-cancer end-points that share common default assumptions and principles. The interpretation of data as indicative of a potential neurotoxic effect involves the evaluation of the validity of the database. There are four principal questions that should be addressed: (1) whether the effects result from exposure; (2) whether the effects are neurotoxicologically significant; (3) whether there is internal consistency between behavioural, physiological, neuro-chemical and morphological end-points; and (4) whether the effects are predictive of what will happen under various conditions. Addressing these issues can provide a useful framework for evaluating either human or animal studies or the weight of evidence for a chemical (Sette & MacPhail, 1992; Health Canada, 1994; Hertel, 1996; IPCS, 1999).

2.3 Examples of chemical-induced neurotoxicity

As can be seen in Table 1, the nervous system is affected by several classes of chemicals found in the environment globally, particu-larly metals, solvents, insecticides and naturally occurring toxins (US NRC, 1992; Spencer et al., 2000). Lead is one of the earliest examples of a neurotoxic chemical with widespread exposure (Gibson, 1904). This metal is widely distributed. Major sources of inorganic lead include industrial emissions, lead-based paints, food, beverages and the burning of leaded gasolines. If exposure occurs at relatively low levels during development, lead can cause a variety of neurobehavioural problems, including learning disorders and altered mental development (Bellinger et al., 1987; Needleman, 1990; Cory-Slechta & Pounds, 1995; Needleman et al., 1996). Over the years, government regulations have been developed to decrease human exposure to lead, and an inter-vention level of 10 µg/dl whole blood has been recommended as a goal (US CDC, 1991; WHO, 1995). While adults appear to be less suscep-tible than children to inorganic lead, occupational exposures to organic lead compounds such as tetraethyl lead have been reported to produce toxic psychosis in adults. Acute solvent intoxication has produced

Table 1. Some examples of human neurotoxicity[a]

Year(s)	Location	Substance[b]	Comments on exposure	Effects[c]	Reference
1904	Australia	Lead	Children exposed to leaded paint	Encephalopathy	Klaassen et al. (1996)
1924	USA	Tetraethyl lead	Occupational exposure	Psychosis	Rosner & Markowitz (1985)
1930	USA	TOCP	Contaminated beverages: more than 50 000 cases	Central/peripheral neuropathy	Spencer et al. (2000)
1930s	Europe	TOCP	Contaminated drug: 60 cases	Central/peripheral neuropathy	Spencer et al. (2000)
1932	USA	Thallium	Contaminated barley	Sensory neuropathy	Spencer et al. (2000)
1937	South Africa	TOCP	Contaminated cooking oil	Central/peripheral neuropathy	Spencer et al. (2000)
1946	England	Tetraethyl lead	Observed in people cleaning gasoline tanks	Encephalopathy	Cassells & Dodds (1946)
1950s	Japan	Methylmercury	Ingestion of contaminated shellfish	Multiple CNS/PNS effects	Spencer et al. (2000)
1950s	France	Diethyltin	Due to medication containing diethyltin diiodide	CNS oedema	Spencer et al. (2000)
1950s	Morocco	Manganese	Miners	Parkinsonian-like syndrome	Spencer et al. (2000)
1950s	Guam	Cycad	Ingestion of plant material	Dementia	Spencer et al. (2000)
1950s	Italy	Carbon disulfide	Occupational exposure	Depression and suicide	Vigliani (1954)
1959	Morocco	TOCP	Contaminated cooking oil	Central/peripheral neuropathy	Spencer et al. (2000)

Table 1 (Contd).

Year(s)	Location	Substance[b]	Comments on exposure	Effects[c]	Reference
1968	Japan	PCBs	Rice oil	Neurodevelopmental cognitive effects	Goetz (1985)
1969	Japan	n-Hexane	Occupational exposure	Central/peripheral neuropathy	Spencer et al. (2000)
1969	USA	Methylmercury	Contaminated grain	Multiple CNS/PNS effects	Pierce et al. (1972)
1971	USA	Hexachlorophene	Contaminated disinfectant	CNS oedema and demyelination	Klaassen et al. (1986)
1971	Iraq	Methylmercury	Contaminated grain seed	Central/peripheral neuropathy	Weiss & Clarkson (1986)
1972	France	Hexachlorophene	Contaminated disinfectant	CNS oedema and demyelination	Martin-Bouyer et al. (1982)
1972–1989	China	3-Nitropropionate	Fungal toxin	Coma followed by spasticity	He et al. (1990)
1973	USA	Methyl n-butyl ketone	Occupational exposure	Central/peripheral neuropathy	Billmaier et al. (1974)
1974–1975	USA	Chlordecone	Occupational exposure	Tremor, hyperexcitability	Spencer et al. (2000)
1975–1977	Germany	n-Hexane and methyl ethyl ketone	25 cases of glue sniffing	Central/peripheral neuropathy	Spencer et al. (2000)
1976	Pakistan	Malathion	2800 people poisoned by impure product	Cholinergic overstimulation	Spencer et al. (2000)

Table 1 (Contd).

Year(s)	Location	Substance[b]	Comments on exposure	Effects[c]	Reference
1979–1980	USA	2-t-Butylazo-2-hydroxy-5-methylhexane (Lucel-7)	Occupational exposure	Central, peripheral and optic neuropathy	Horan et al. (1985)
1980s	USA	MPTP	Illicit drug	Parkinson's-like effect	Kopin & Markey (1988)
1981	Spain	Toxic oil	Contaminated cooking oil	Peripheral neuropathy	Altenkirch et al. (1988)
1983–1984	USA	Vitamin B6	Excessive intake	Sensory neuropathy	Spencer et al. (2000)
1985	USA and Canada	Aldicarb	Contaminated melons	Cholinergic overstimulation	Anon (1986)
1987	Canada	Domoic acid	Contaminated mussels	Sensory and CNS degeneration	Perl et al. (1990)
1988	Sri Lanka	TOCP	Contaminated oil	Peripheral neuropathy	Spencer et al. (2000)
1996	Japan	Sarin	Terrorist attack	Cholinergic overstimulation	Yokoyama et al. (1998)

[a] Adapted from US NRC (1992).
[b] PCBs = polychlorinated biphenyls; MPTP = 1-methyl-4-phenyl-1,2,3,6-tetrahydropyridine; TOCP = tri-o-cresylphosphate.
[c] CNS = central nervous system; PNS = peripheral nervous system.

13

dementia, but this is relatively rare (Cassells & Dodds, 1946; Arlien-Søborg, 1992).

Organic mercury compounds are potent neurotoxic substances and have caused a number of human poisonings, with symptoms and signs of vision, speech and coordination impairments (Chang, 1980; Chang & Verity, 1995; Myers & Davidson, 1998). One major incident of human exposure occurred in the mid-1950s when a chemical plant near Minamata Bay, Japan, discharged mercury sulfate used as a catalyst for the synthesis of acetaldehyde into the wastewater from the plant as part of waste sludge. The discharged mercury was converted to methyl-mercury sulfide by microbial organisms, and an epidemic of methyl-mercury poisoning developed when the local inhabitants consumed contaminated fish and shellfish. Affected children displayed a progres-sive neurological disturbance resembling cerebral palsy and manifested other neurological problems as well. In 1971, an epidemic occurred in Iraq from methylmercury used as a fungicide to treat grain (US OTA, 1990). A syndrome with such neurological features as tremor and such behavioural symptoms as anxiety, irritability and pathological shyness is seen in people exposed to elemental mercury.

Manganese is an essential dietary substance for normal body func-tioning, yet exposure to large amounts of manganese can be neurotoxic, producing a dyskinetic motor syndrome similar to Parkinson's disease (Cook et al., 1974; Chu et al., 1995). Exposed manganese miners in several countries have suffered from "manganese madness," charac-terized by hallucinations, emotional instability and numerous neuro-logical problems. Long-term manganese toxicity produces muscle rigidity and a shuffling gait similar to that seen in patients with Parkin-son's disease (Politis et al., 1980).

Another example of a Parkinsonian-like syndrome is the move-ment disorder observed in drug abusers who intravenously injected 1-methyl-4-phenyl-1,2,3,6-tetrahydropyridine (MPTP) (Langston et al., 1983). MPTP is a by-product of a meperidine derivative sold illicitly as "synthetic heroin."

Organic solvents are encountered frequently in occupational settings (Dick, 1995), and some are reported to produce clinical neuro-psychological and neurological effects (White, 1995). Most solvents are volatile — i.e., they can be converted from a liquid to a vapour and readily inhaled by the worker. Some solvents, such as carbon disulfide, can, at high doses, produce specific neurotoxicological effects, including toxic polyneuropathy and a syndrome consisting of tremor and neuropsychological deficits in motor, affective, visuospatial, attention, executive and memory function (Seppäläinen & Haltia, 1980; White, 1995). Furthermore, repeated exposure to organic solvents is suspected of producing chronic encephalopathy (Arlien-Søborg, 1992; IPCS, 1996b). Workers exposed to methyl *n*-butyl ketone (an ink solvent and cleaning agent) displayed peripheral neuropathy involving sensory and motor changes of the hands and feet (Dick, 1995). Some solvents, including ethers, ketones, alcohols and various combinations, are commonly used in glues, cements and paints and can be neurotoxic when inhaled (Altenkirch, 1982; Altenkirch et al., 1988). Repeated abuse of such solvents can lead to permanent neurological effects due to severe and permanent loss of nerve cells (US OTA, 1990). Case–control studies have also shown that a history of organic solvent exposure may be associated with increased risk of deficits similar to those seen with Alzheimer's disease (Kukull et al., 1995).

Pesticides are one of the most commonly encountered classes of neurotoxic substances. They can include insecticides (used to control insects), fungicides (for blight and mildew), rodenticides (for rodents, such as rats, mice and gophers) and herbicides (to control weeds) (Hayes, 1991). Active ingredients are combined with so-called inert substances to make thousands of different pesticide formulations. Workers who are overexposed to organophosphate pesticides may display obvious signs and symptoms of poisoning, including tremors, weakness, ataxia, visual disturbances and short-term memory loss (Ecobichon & Joy, 1982; Abou-Donia, 1995). The organophosphate insecticides have neurotoxic properties and account for approximately 40% of registered pesticides in the USA. Delayed neurotoxicity can be seen as a result of exposure to certain organophosphate pesticides, producing loss of motor function and an associated neuropathology (Ecobichon & Joy, 1982). Organophosphate and carbamate insecticides are known to interfere with a specific enzyme, acetylcholinesterase (AChE) (Davis & Richardson, 1980; Abou-Donia, 1995; Metcalf, 1995). Neuropathy has also been reported following consumption of non-pesticide organophosphates, such as tri-*o*-cresylphosphate (TOCP). Other classes of pesticides, including the organochlorines (Cannon et al., 1978; Woolley, 1995) and pyrethroids (Clark, 1995), may produce signs of functional neurotoxicity. A number of reports have noted that many cases of human poisonings due to the ingestion or absorption of neurotoxic pesticides go unreported. This is especially true in developing countries, where up to 45% of pesticide poisoning cases occur in young children (WHO, 2000).

Neurotoxicities in humans, domestic livestock and poultry associated with fungal toxins (mycotoxins) have been well documented (Wyllie & Morehouse, 1978; Aibara, 1986; Kurata, 1990; Ludolph & Spencer, 1995). An example of human exposure to fungal toxins is *Claviceps purpurea-* or *C. paspali-*infected wheat, barley and oats used for bread and as a dietary supplement for livestock. These fungal toxins are notorious for producing the gangrenous and convulsive forms of the disease known as "ergotism" (Bove, 1970). Fungi in the family Clavicipitaceae produce ergot alkaloids, which have neurotropic, uterotonic and vasoconstrictive activities, possibly related to their sympathomimetic effects. Other fungi associated with ergot-like syndromes in livestock include *Acremonium lolii* (Gallagher et al., 1984) and *A. coenophialum* (Thompson & Porter, 1990). Cyclopiazonic acid (CPA) is an indole tetramic acid produced by *Aspergillus flavus, A. oryzae, Penicillium cyclopium* and *P. camemberti.* This mycotoxin is suspected of causing "kodua poisoning" in humans who consumed kodo millet seed in India (Rao & Husain, 1985). *Fusarium moniliforme* is a common fungal infection in corn (Bacon et al., 1992) and is directly related to a neurotoxic syndrome in horses known as equine leukoencephalopathy. The fungal metabolite 3-nitropropionic acid has poisoned both people and grazing animals. In northern China, fungi growing on sugarcane stored over winter for the New Year Festival were responsible for at least 885 poisonings and 88 deaths over the period 1972–1989 (He et al., 1995). Nitropropionic acid is produced by various fungi of the genus *Arthrinium*, as well as *Aspergillus* and *Penicillium*, and causes selective neuronal loss in the striatum (Fu et al., 1995).

Many bacteria have been shown to produce toxins that affect the nervous system, including cholera toxin, diphtheria toxin, botulinum neurotoxin and tetanus toxin (Simpson et al., 1995). Many venoms produced by spiders and snakes also affect the nervous system (Tu, 1995). Neurotoxins have also been found in many aquatic species, including tetrodotoxin (puffer fish), saxitoxin (paralytic shellfish) and ciguatoxin in *Gambierdiscus toxicus*, a dinoflagellate. An outbreak of toxic encephalopathy caused by eating mussels contaminated with domoic acid, an excitotoxin, was reported in North America (Perl et al., 1990). Neurotoxicity has been reported in several individuals exposed to *Pfisteria piscicida* (Glasgow et al., 1995), a newly recognized species of toxic dinoflagellates. Examples of toxins in food include buckthorn toxin in the fruit of *Karwinska humboldtiana*, which produces a progressive peripheral neuropathy, and cassava, which produces a cyanogenic glycoside associated with tropical ataxic neuropathy (Mitchell & Shaw, 1999).

2.4 Definitions and critical concepts in neurotoxicology

This section defines the key terms and concepts often used in neurotoxicity risk assessment and sets the stage for subsequent chapters (O'Donoghue, 1994).

2.4.1 Neurotoxicity versus adverse effects

Neurotoxicity has been defined as an adverse change in the structure or function of the central nervous system (CNS) and/or peripheral nervous system (PNS) following exposure to a chemical (natural or synthetic) or physical agent (Tilson, 1990b; ECETOC, 1992; Ladefoged et al., 1995). The Nordic Council of Ministers (Johnsen et al., 1992) defined neurotoxicity as the capability of inducing adverse effects in the CNS, peripheral nerves or sense organs. A chemical is considered to be a neurotoxicant if it induces a consistent pattern of neural dysfunction or lesion in the nervous system (Johnsen et al., 1992).

Disagreement exists among toxicologists as to what constitutes an "adverse change." One commonly accepted definition of adverse effect is a treatment-related alteration from baseline that diminishes an organism's ability to survive, reproduce or adapt to the environment (ECETOC, 1992; Ladefoged et al., 1995; US EPA, 1998a). The term "adverse" may also be considered in the toxicological sense, connoting a detrimental change in structure and/or function of the nervous system (ECETOC, 1992; US EPA, 1998a). The OECD/IPCS project on the harmonization of hazard/risk assessment terminology (OECD/IPCS, 2001) defines an adverse effect as a change in morphology, physiology, growth, development or life span of an organism that results in an impairment of functional capacity, an impairment of the capacity to compensate for additional stress or an increase in susceptibility to other environmental influences.

Structural neurotoxic effects are defined as neuroanatomical changes occurring at any level of nervous system organization. Functional changes are defined as neurochemical, neurophysiological or behavioural effects. Functional neurotoxic effects include adverse changes in somatic/autonomic, sensory, motor and cognitive function.

2.4.2 Direct versus indirect effects

Chemically induced neurotoxic effects may be direct (i.e., due to an agent or its metabolites acting directly on sites in the nervous system) or indirect (i.e., due to agents or metabolites that produce their effects primarily by interacting with sites outside the nervous system) (ECETOC, 1992; O'Donoghue, 1994; Ladefoged et al., 1995). Direct neurotoxic effects are viewed with a high degree of concern in risk assessment. Indirect effects are more difficult to evaluate. It is often difficult to differentiate between direct and indirect effects, especially when the mechanisms of neurotoxicity are not known (Ladefoged et al., 1995). Consideration of dose is also an important factor. It is also problematic that some functional tests (i.e., behavioural changes) may be indirectly affected by systemic toxicity (ECETOC, 1992; Ladefoged et al., 1995; US EPA, 1998a). Before functional changes can be considered to be neurotoxic effects, the extent to which gross toxicity, loss of body weight or alterations in normal metabolic processes of the body may have been compromised should be determined. Indirect effects of chemicals on the nervous system should be assessed in terms of the type and severity of change and the dose–response relationship of those effects relative to other measures of toxicity.

2.4.3 Primary versus secondary effects

A potentially confusing factor is that neurotoxic effects can be produced either by chemicals that do not require metabolism prior to interacting with their sites in the nervous system (i.e., primary neuro-toxic agents) or by chemicals that require metabolism prior to inter-acting with their sites in the nervous system (i.e., secondary neurotoxic agents) (O'Donoghue, 1994). Demonstrated primary or secondary neurotoxic agents should be considered with a high degree of concern.

2.4.4 *Transient versus persistent effects*

Chemically induced effects resulting in a slowly reversible or in an irreversible persistent change in the structure or function of the organism are viewed with a particularly high degree of concern in risk assessment. Such effects are viewed differently from transient, acute effects of chemicals. It has been argued (ECETOC, 1992; Johnsen et al., 1992) that reversible functional or behavioural effects not associated with permanent morphological alterations are not necessarily neurotoxic, although they may have adverse consequences. Others (Ladefoged et al., 1995) argue that the requirement for morphological changes may be problematic. For example, morphological changes may be transient or develop slowly. In addition, it may not be possible to accurately determine where the structural damage occurred without extensive neuropathological examination. These authors suggest that transient effects should be judged based on the severity of the effect and the context in which the chemical is used. For example, transient changes in motor performance that could affect the operation of dangerous equipment in an occupational setting would be viewed with a high degree of concern. An evaluation of the relevance of the doses at which effects occur would normally take place during the exposure assessment phase of the risk assessment process.

2.4.5 *Compensation*

The nervous system is known for its reserve capacity (Tilson & Mitchell, 1983; Weiss, 1990) and for its ability to compensate for neurotoxic insult. There are, however, limits to the capacity for adaptation; when these limits are exceeded, further exposure could lead to frank manifestations of neurotoxicity at the structural or functional level. In addition, it is now clear that neurotoxic insults may be hidden by compensatory mechanisms. The concern is that the brain, once damaged, may show decreased capacity to withstand subsequent insult (Weiss, 1990). Reduced ability to compensate may be revealed experimentally after such environmental challenges as neuroactive drugs, certain testing conditions, stress, aging or even socioeconomic conditions (Bellinger & Matthews, 1998). Evidence of diminished ability to compensate is viewed with a high degree of concern.

2.5 Assumptions in neurotoxicity risk assessment

There are a number of unknowns in the extrapolation of data from animal studies to humans (ECETOC, 1992; Johnsen et al., 1992; US EPA, 1998a).

It is generally assumed that an agent that produces detectable adverse neurotoxic effects in experimental animal studies will pose a potential hazard to humans. This assumption is based on the comparisons of data for known human neurotoxicants (Kimmel et al., 1990; Chang & Dyer, 1995; Spencer et al., 2000), which indicate that experimental animal data are frequently predictive of a neurotoxic effect in humans. However, there are notable differences between animals and humans in sensitivity to some neurotoxicants. For example, MPTP is highly neurotoxic to humans and other primates, but not to rats (Snyder & D'Amato, 1986). Although most clinical neurotoxicity signs can be reproduced in animal models using rodents, this is not always the case. Therefore, it may be difficult to determine which will be the most appropriate species in terms of predicting the specific types of effects seen in humans. The fact that every species may not react in the same way may be due to species-specific differences in maturation of the nervous system, differences in timing of exposure or biochemical and pharmacokinetic factors. There are also basic structural differences (e.g., pigmentation of substantia nigra) that may underlie species differences.

Issues concerning the extrapolation of data from animals to humans in neurotoxicology have been reviewed by McMillan & Owens (1995). A number of default assumptions are made that are generally applied in the absence of data on the relevance of effects to potential human risk. Default assumptions should not be applied indiscriminately. All available mechanistic and pharmacokinetic data should be considered first (Andersen et al., 1991). If these data indicate that an alternative assumption is appropriate or obviate the need for applying an assumption, such information should be used in risk assessment. For example, research using rats may determine that the neurotoxicity of a chemical is caused by a metabolite. If subsequent research finds that the chemical is metabolized to a lesser degree or not at all in humans, then this information should be used in formulating the default assumptions.

It is also assumed that behavioural, neurophysiological, neuro-chemical and neuroanatomical manifestations are of concern. Neuro-toxicity is generally seen as a continuum of signs and effects, which depend on the chemical, the dose and the duration of exposure (Johnsen et al., 1992). Laboratory studies in volunteers and experi-mental animal studies frequently use exposure levels that are higher than the average environmental levels. In the past, the tendency has been to consider only neuropathological changes as end-points of concern, although this is no longer considered valid (Ladefoged et al., 1995). Based on data from agents known to be human neurotoxicants (Anger, 1990a,b; Kimmel et al., 1990; Chang & Dyer, 1995), there is usually at least one experimental species that mimics the types of effects seen in humans; in other species tested, however, the type of neurotoxic effect may be different or absent. A biologically significant change in animals is considered indicative of an agent's potential for disrupting the structure or function of the human nervous system.

Finally, in the absence of data to the contrary, the most sensitive species will be used to estimate human risk. This is based on the assumption that humans are as sensitive as the most sensitive animal species tested. This assumption is made to provide a conservative estimate of sensitivity for added protection to the public. Like other non-cancer end-points, it is assumed that there is a non-linear dose–response relationship for neurotoxicants. Threshold effects for neuro-toxicity can be difficult to observe empirically (OECD/IPCS, 2001).

2.6   Criteria for quality of data used in risk assessment

The value of test methods for quantitative neurotoxicity risk assessment is related to a number of criteria, including demonstration of (1) sensitivity to the kinds of neurobehavioural impairment produced by chemicals (e.g., ability to detect a difference between exposed and non-exposed populations); (2) specificity for neurotoxic chemical effects (e.g., no undue responsiveness to a host of other non-chemical factors) and specificity for the neurobiological end-point believed to be measured by the test method; (3) adequate reliability (consistency of measurement over time); and (4) validity (concordance with other behavioural, physiological, biochemical or anatomic measures of neurotoxicity). It is also important to show graded amounts of change as a function of exposure level, absorbed dose or body burden (dose–response). For representative classes or subclasses of chemicals that are active in the CNS or PNS, it is important to be able to identify single effects or patterns of impairment across several tests or functional domains that are reasonably consistent from study to study. Test methods should also be amenable to the development of a procedurally similar counterpart that can be used to assess homologous measures in humans and animals. Data that provide information on mechanism of action are of particular value in risk assessment.

2.6.1 Sensitivity

Individual neurotoxicological tests and test batteries have detected differences between exposed and non-exposed populations in epidemiological and laboratory studies. Effects have been detected by some neurobiological methods at concentrations at which effects were not detected by other methods. While the overall sensitivity of neurobiological methods is sufficient to be useful in neurotoxicity risk assessment, some methods are notably insensitive across several chemical classes, while the sensitivity of other tests varies according to the spectrum of neurotoxic effects of the chemical or drug. Sensitivity is sometimes negatively correlated with reliability (Ray, 1997); selecting for end-points that show little change over time may also select for tests that are not sensitive to neurotoxic insult.

2.6.2 Specificity

There are two kinds of specificity in the assessment of neurotoxicity. Chemical specificity refers to the ability of a test to reflect chemical effects and to be relatively resistant to the influence of unrelated chemicals or of non-chemical variables. The second type of specificity refers to the ability of a test method to measure changes in a single function (e.g., dexterity) or a restricted number of functions, rather than a broad range of functions (attention, reasoning, dexterity and vision). The neurobiological expression of neurotoxicity is a function of the joint interaction of ongoing nervous system processes with the chemical substance and with biopsychosocial variables that also influence nervous system activity. In laboratory exposure studies, numerous environmental, behavioural and biological variables can influence the type or magnitude of neurotoxic effects of chemical agents and drugs (MacPhail, 1990).

2.6.3 *Reliability/validity*

Reliability refers to the ability of a given test to produce closely similar results when administered more than once over a period of time or in similar populations. Reliability is meaningful only with respect to the measurement of functions that would not be expected to change significantly over the time period. Validity refers to the concordance of several different types of measures, which suggests a biologically plausible effect, rather than a random pattern.

2.6.4 *Dose–response*

Dose is the total amount of a substance administered to, taken in or absorbed by an organism (OECD/IPCS, 2001). A dose–response relationship may be defined as a link between the amount of a chemical or biological agent taken in or absorbed by a system and the resulting quantified change developed in that system (OECD/IPCS, 2001). Both exposure concentrations and biological concentrations should be measured whenever possible. Dose–response relationships have been observed in both field and laboratory studies. A review of over 50 human exposure studies involving organic solvents found that neurobehavioural impairment generally occurred at mean concentrations higher than those associated with irritation, although there was often overlap among the irritant and impairment concentration ranges (Dick, 1988). Defining neurotoxic dose–response relationships in humans decreases the uncertainties of extrapolation from animal data and allows a more accurate risk assessment.

A further complication in dose–response extrapolation is that low concentrations of chemicals may appear to improve performance as measured by some neurobehavioural tests, while higher doses are more likely to impair performance. Improved performance does not necessarily indicate the absence of neurotoxicity; both increases and decreases in neurobehavioural performance may result from deleterious chemical interactions with neurons. Dose–response extrapolation is further complicated by the observation that facilitative or impairment effects within a given dosage range may occur at some parameters of the test stimulus or aspects of the response (response rate dependent), but not at others (Altmann et al., 1991). Therefore, dose extrapolations are more difficult when there is uncertainty about the shape of the dose–response function (biphasic, linear, etc.) at the relevant test stimulus and response parameters.

The risk assessment process utilizing animal data often involves extrapolation from the effects of high doses in animals to predict the effects of chronic low-dose exposure in humans. With data from laboratory studies of humans in a risk assessment, however, the extrapolation may also be in the other direction, from very low dose laboratory exposure to predict the effects of chronic exposure at higher (but still low) concentrations in the environment and workplace. Low-to high-dose extrapolation within the same species may require different assumptions and risk assessment procedures. Although high-dose human exposures have occurred in accidents, those data are primarily descriptive in nature and cannot easily be used in a quantitative risk extrapolation process. However, low-dose laboratory data may be combined with data from epidemiological studies of persons exposed to higher concentrations.

3. BASIC PRINCIPLES FOR NEUROTOXICITY RISK ASSESSMENT

3.1 Neurobiological principles

3.1.1 Structure of the nervous system

The nervous system consists of the brain and spinal cord (CNS), peripheral nerves, and the organs of special sense (Raine, 1994). The PNS is divided into the somatic (motor and sensory) and the autonomic nervous system. Within the nervous system, there exist predominantly two general types of cells — nerve cells (neurons) and neuroglial cells. Neurons have many of the same structures found in every cell of the body. They are unique, however, in that they have axons and dendrites, extensions of the neuron along which nerve impulses travel. The structure of the neuron consists of a cell body, 10–100 μm in diameter, containing a nucleus and organelles for the synthesis of various components necessary for the cell's functioning. Numerous branch patterns of elongated processes, the dendrites, emanate from the cell body and increase the neuronal surface area available to receive inputs from other sources. The axon is a process specialized for the conduction of nerve impulses away from the cell towards the terminal synapses and eventually towards other cells (neurons, muscle cells or gland cells). The axons of sensory cells can conduct nerve impulses towards the cell body. In general, the length of the axon is tens to thousands of times greater than the cell body diameter. For example, the cell body whose processes innervate the muscles in the human foot is found in the spinal cord at the level of the middle back. Neurons are responsible for the reception, integration, transmission and storage of information (Raine, 1994). Certain nerve cells are specialized to respond to particular stimuli. For example, chemoreceptors in the mouth and nose send information about taste and smell to the brain. Cutaneous receptors in the skin are involved in the sensation of pressure, pain, heat, cold and touch. In the retina, the rods and cones sense light.

Many, but not all, axons are surrounded by the layers of membrane from the cytoplasmic process of neuroglial cells. These layers are called myelin sheaths and are composed mostly of lipid. In the PNS, the myelin sheaths are formed by Schwann cells, while in the CNS, the sheaths are formed by the oligodendroglia. In the PNS, there is a one to one relationship between the Schwann cell and the underlying axon (Webster, 1975), while in the CNS, the oligodendrocyte produces multiple cellular extensions that can form myelin internodes on multiple axons (Chang & Dyer, 1995). In each case, only one segment is produced for a given axon. Each glial cell covers only a short length of any one axon; thus, the entire length of any one axon is ensheathed in myelin by numerous glial cells. There are periodic interruptions along the axons between adjacent myelin internodes; termed nodes of Ranvier, these short intervals where axons are not enveloped by myelin are vital for normal nervous system function. In unmyelinated axons, a nerve impulse must travel in a continuous sequential manner down the entire length of the axon. The presence of myelin accelerates the nerve impulse by up to 100 times by allowing the impulse to jump from one node to the next in a process called "saltatory conduction." Saltatory conduction is more rapid and requires less energy than conduction in unmyelinated axons. Thus, myelin serves to increase the efficiency of the nervous system by facilitating conduction, yet conserving metabolic energy.

In addition to the oligodendrocytes and Schwann cells, the brain contains other neuroglia, the astrocytes and the microglia. Astrocytes and microglia are usually considered because of their response to injury, but both glial cells also play a significant role in the formation and functioning of the normal brain. Only a brief accounting of some of the many features of the astrocytes and microglia will be presented here. The morphological response of glia to injury is presented in chapter 5.

Microglial cell numbers have been estimated to comprise between 5 and 20% of total brain glia (e.g., Kreutzberg, 1987). They are highly ramified cells with a small amount of perinuclear cytoplasm and a small dense and heterochromatic nucleus. These small microglia have a complex plasma membrane, containing a large number of receptor and adhesion molecules as well as enzymatic activities, and can be distinguished from other glial cells by their surface immunophenotype. Microglia are located outside of the vascular basement membrane, yet their cytoplasmic processes are found intermingled with the layer of astrocytic foot processes (Lassmann et al., 1991). They are distributed throughout the normal CNS; however, regional differences have been reported in mouse brain, with the highest densities in the hippocampus, olfactory telencephalon, basal ganglia and substantia nigra (Lawson et al., 1990). Microglia in the grey matter tend to be profusely ramified, with processes extending in multiple directions, while cells in the white matter often align their cytoplasmic extensions in parallel to nerve fibre bundles. While the function of resting microglia is not known, it has become evident that resting microglia rapidly undergo morphological changes in response to injury. These cells form part of an intrinsic immune complex in the nervous system due to their capacity to phagocytose and to release several immunomodulatory substances.

The radial glial cell is generally recognized as the first subtype of astroglia to appear in the brain (Misson et al., 1991). During development, radial glial cells play a crucial role in the construction of the nervous system by providing scaffolding for the migrating neurons and participating in the formation of diverse glial cell lineages (Rakic, 1971, 1972). The gliophilic migration of neurons is evident during the formation of the cerebellum (Rakic, 1971), the neocortex (Rakic, 1972) and the hippocampus (Eckenhoff & Rakic, 1991). This association during the formation of brain regions is critically dependent upon cell–cell interactions between the neurons and glia as well as signalling from the extracellular environment. Once neuronal migration is completed, the radial glia can give rise to astrocytes in both the grey and white matter of the brain and spinal cord. There are three main types of astrocytes according to their spatial organization: (1) radial astrocytes, which are disposed in a plane perpendicular to the axis of the ventricles and span the whole thickness of the white matter; (2) fibrous, non-radial astrocytes, which send processes in multiple directions and do not contact pia mater; and (3) protoplasmic astrocytes, which have short ramified crimped processes located in the grey matter.

Glial cells, and particularly astrocytes, structurally envelop synapses in a way that would allow for the interception of transmitter molecules that overflow from the synaptic cleft. They are also equipped with the transport systems and enzymes that are necessary to degrade most known neurotransmitters (Chang & Dyer, 1995). Astrocytes can express a multiplicity of cell surface receptors. They can respond to amino acids, amines, peptides, purines and prostaglandins. The role for such receptors is a major topic of current research efforts. Astrocytes have an essential role in maintaining the ionic balance of the neuronal extracellular space. In astrocytes, transient cytosolic calcium changes produce several immediate, intermediate and long-term changes in glial structure and function. Thus, astrocytes exert a dynamic influence on the development and functioning of the nervous system via multiple mechanisms.

3.1.2 Transport processes

All types of cells are required to transport proteins and other molecular components from their site of synthesis near the nucleus to the various other sites of usage in the cell. In the nervous system, axonal transport is the process by which the neuron replenishes components of the axon and the nerve terminal. The cell body of the neuron must maintain the functions normally associated with its own support, as well as provide continuous support of its various processes. Proteins and other macromolecules destined for axonal transport are either quickly routed into the axon or stored in a cell body compartment for later export into the neurites. Organelles are targeted and delivered to specific domains within the axon, such as the axolemma (axonal membrane), nodes of Ranvier and presynaptic terminals (for review, see Hammerschlag & Stone, 1982; Kelly, 1985). Material is returned to the cell body as a signalling process, for degradation or reutilization. This interneuronal traffic, including the molecular motors that drive the organelles along axonal substrates, comprises the components of the process of axonal transport (for review, see Hammerschlag et al., 1994). Fast transport is the process by which the neuron provides newly synthesized material necessary to maintain the axonal and nerve terminal membranes. Cytoskeletal elements and soluble proteins are transported down the axon by slow axoplasmic flow, providing for the continual renewal of the structural proteins comprising the neurofilament and microtubule network of the axon (Lasek & Brady, 1982; Lasek et al., 1984). Once reaching the nerve terminals, much of the slowly transported material is rapidly degraded, presumably by specific calcium-activated proteases (Garner, 1988; Sahenk & Lasek, 1988), while much of the material transported by fast transport returns to the cell body, either for degradation or for restoration and reuse (for review, see Kristersson, 1987). The anterograde movement of membrane-bound organelles such as synaptic vesicles, mitochondria and lysosomes is associated with the microtubule-activated ATPase kinesin (Brady, 1985, 1991; Cyr & Brady, 1992). Material is driven along microtubules in a retrograde direction by the microtubule-associated ATPase dynein. While most of this material is the result of a reversal or turnaround at the nerve ending, extracellular material can be taken up at the terminals by endocytosis and retrogradely transported. Nerve terminal endocytosis can retrieve both endogenous substances, such as nerve growth factor, and harmful substances, such as neurotropic viruses, and transport them to the cell body.

3.1.3 Ion channels

The excitable membrane of the nerve cell is particularly sensitive to changes in intra- and extracellular ion concentrations. Thus, a tight regulation of intraneuronal ion concentrations is required, which is accomplished by a relatively impermeable membrane, various ion pumps, intracellular ion binding sites and a variety of specific ion channels. These channels may be voltage sensitive, directly associated with membrane receptors or linked to a cascade of intracellular signals (i.e., second messengers). One critical process for regulation is the maintenance of calcium homeostasis. Intracytoplasmic calcium homeostasis is maintained by calcium binding proteins, voltage-sensitive plasma membrane calcium channels, plasmalemma calcium ATPase pumping calcium ions across the membrane, plasma membrane sodium–calcium exchanges and intracellular calcium storage organelles (e.g., mitrochondria and endoplasmic reticulum). An alteration in any one of these processes resulting in altered calcium homeostasis can lead to cytotoxicity in the neuron. For example, neuronal toxicity induced by glutamate and other excitatory amino acids (EAAs) is characterized by acute swelling of the dendrites and cell body subsequent to a slower calcium-dependent neuronal degeneration (Choi, 1988).

The axonal membrane is semipermeable to positively and negatively charged ions (mostly potassium, sodium and chloride) within and outside of the axon. There are several enzyme systems that maintain an ionic balance that changes following depolarization of the membrane (Davies, 1968; Hille & Catterall, 1994). This is maintained only by the continual active transport of ions across the membrane, which requires an expenditure of energy. The nerve impulse is a travelling wave of depolarization normally originating from the cell body; however, in sensory neurons, it originates at the terminal receptive end of specialized axons (Davies, 1968). The wave is continued by openings in the membrane that allow ions to rush into the axon. This sudden change in the charge across the axon's membrane is the nerve impulse, which spreads down the axon from one length to the next length of membrane. It continues in this fashion until it reaches the synaptic terminal regions. There are a number of varieties of membrane channels (e.g., calcium) that rapidly open and close during impulse generation; the common ones are the sodium and potassium channels. They are very small and allow only ions of a certain size to pass. Several classes of drugs (e.g., local anaesthetics) and natural toxins (e.g., tetrodotoxin) inhibit nerve impulse conduction by blocking these channels. The activity of ion channels can be modified by cellular metabolic reactions, including protein phosphorylation, various ions that act as blockers, and toxins, poisons and drugs. If the flow of ions across the cell membrane is changed, the transmission of information between nerve cells will be altered.

Membrane ion channels are important targets in various diseases, such as the autoimmune neurological disorders myasthenia gravis and Lambert-Eaton syndrome. Both are thought to result from the action of specific antibodies interfering with channel function. Cystic fibrosis is thought to involve a genetic defect in the control of a certain type of chloride channel.

3.1.4 Neurotransmission

The terminal branches of the axon end in small enlargements called synaptic "boutons." It is from these boutons that chemical messengers will be released in order to communicate with the target cell at the point of interaction, the synapse (Erulkar, 1994). When the nerve impulse reaches the terminal branches of the axon, it depolarizes the synaptic boutons. This depolarization causes the release of the chemical messengers (neurotransmitters and neuromodulators) stored in vesicles in the axon terminal (Willis & Grossman, 1973). Classical neurotransmitters include serotonin, dopamine, acetylcholine, norepinephrine, glutamic acid and γ-aminobutyric acid (GABA) and are typically released by one neuron into the synaptic cleft, where they bind to receptors on the postsynaptic membrane. Others include the amino acids glycine and aspartate, as well as various purines. Neuropeptides may travel long distances through the bloodstream to receptors on distant nerve cells or in other tissues. Following depolarization, the amount of secretion is dependent on the number of nerve impulses that reach the synaptic bouton, i.e., the degree of depolarization. The chemical messengers diffuse across the synaptic cleft or into the intraneuronal space and bind to receptors on adjacent nerve cells or effector organs, thus triggering biochemical events that lead to electrical excitation or inhibition.

When information is transmitted from nerves to muscle fibres via the neurotransmitter acetylcholine, the point of interaction is called the neuromuscular junction, and the interaction leads to contraction or relaxation of the muscle. When the target is a gland cell, the interaction leads to secretion. Synaptic transmission between neurons is slightly more complicated but still dependent on the opening and closing of ion channels in the membrane. The binding of the messenger to the receptor of the receiving cell can lead to either the excitation or inhibition of the target cell. At an excitatory synapse, the neurotransmitter–receptor interaction leads to an opening in certain ion-specific channels. The charged ions that move through these opened chambers carry a current that serves to depolarize the cell membranes. At inhibitory synapses, the interaction leads to an opening in a different type of ion-specific channel, which produces an increase in the level of polarization (hyperpolarization). The sum of all the depolarizing and hyperpolarizing currents determines the transmembrane potential; when a threshold level of depolarization is reached at the axon's initial segment, a nerve impulse is generated and begins to travel down the axon.

The duration of neurotransmitter action is primarily a function of the length of time it remains in the synaptic cleft. This duration is very short due to specialized enzymes that quickly remove the transmitter either by degrading it or by reuptake systems that transport it back into the synaptic bouton. A toxic substance may disrupt this process in several different ways. It is important that the duration of the effect of synaptically released chemical messengers be limited. Some neurotoxicants (e.g., cholinesterase-inhibiting organophosphorus pesticides) inhibit the enzyme AChE, which serves to terminate the effect of the neurotransmitter (acetylcholine) on its target. The result is an overstimulation of the target cell. Other substances, particularly biological toxins, are able to interact with the receptor molecule and mimic the action of the neurotransmitter. Some toxic substances, like neuroactive pharmaceuticals, may interfere with the synthesis of a particular neurotransmitter, while others may block the neurotransmitter's access to its receptor molecule or cause excess release.

3.1.5 Metabolism

The CNS has a very high metabolic rate, and, unlike other organs, the brain depends almost entirely on glucose as a source of energy and raw material for the synthesis of other molecules (Damstra & Bondy, 1980; Clarke & Sokoloff, 1994). The necessary continuous supply of oxygen is dependent upon replenishment by the circulation, as only a minimal amount of oxygen is stored in the brain relative to the demands. In order to provide the necessary supply of oxygen, the blood flowing through the brain is a considerable proportion of the total cardiac output, approximately 15%. Energy metabolism is not the only requirement for oxygen in the brain. A part of oxygen consumption is contributed towards the formation of various oxidases and hydroxylases critical in the synthesis and metabolism of a number of neurotransmitters. A significant proportion of brain energy is required for the processes of excitation, conduction and subsequent neurotransmission. Most of the ATP produced in the brain is required to restore the ionic gradients of the membrane constantly altered by synaptic transmission.

The brain has only a limited ability to oxidize substances other than glucose. Glucose utilization in the brain has been examined using 2-[^{14}C]deoxyglucose. A differential level of energy demand can be seen in distinct brain regions, and interference with glucose metabolism can affect numerous regions, including the cerebral cortex, cerebellum and hippocampus. Energy demands of the brain and the required blood flow vary as a function of age, health status or drug state. Animal data suggest that cerebral oxygen consumption is low at birth and rises during the period of cerebral growth and development, reaching a maximal level at maturation of each brain region.

3.1.6 Blood–brain and blood–nerve barriers

The entry, distribution and exit of chemicals from the PNS and CNS are influenced by a variety of morphological and biochemical specializations (Neuwelt, 1989; Pardridge, 1998). Most blood-borne nutrients and xenobiotics enter the extracellular space of nervous system structures by passing through or between adjacent endothelial cells of nearby capillaries. In the PNS, the extracellular fluid drains into the lymphatic circulation. In the brain and spinal cord, the extracellular fluid drains into the cerebral ventricles and subarachnoid space, where it joins the cerebrospinal fluid (CSF). In humans, CSF exits the brain and enters the venous circulation primarily by passing from the subarachnoid space through the arachnoid villi into the superior sagittal sinus. Thus, the exit of many exogenous and endogenous (i.e., the products of neuronal metabolism) materials from the extracellular space is mediated by bulk flow of the extracellular and cerebrospinal fluids.

In the CNS, capillaries serving most of the brain and spinal cord are composed of endothelial cells connected by circumferential tight junctions. These tight junctions limit the diffusion of most materials into (and out of) the extracellular space and are the major anatomical component of the blood–brain barrier (BBB). Although highly lipophilic materials can pass from the luminal to the abluminal surface of the endothelial cells, the transcellular movement of many other materials requires the participation of some kind of transport mechanism. The transcellular passage of iron, ions, glucose, fatty acids, thyroid hormones, nucleosides, low-density lipoproteins and large neutral and basic amino acids across the cerebral endothelial cell all involve a transport mechanism. The entry and/or distribution of several neurotoxicants (e.g., mercury, manganese) in the CNS may be influenced by one of these transport systems (Aschner, 1996; Malecki et al., 1999).

Several sites in the brain are served by capillaries that lack BBB properties. These sites are all located at the mid-sagittal surface of the cerebral ventricles and are termed circumventricular organs (CVOs). The absence of BBB properties at these sites enables free exchange of materials between the blood, CNS extracellular space and CSF. Thus, these brain regions can receive solutes from the blood and release secretory products into the blood and CSF. The CVOs include the choroid plexuses (which secrete CSF), pineal gland, neurohypophysis, the organum vasculosum of the lamina terminalis, median eminence, subfornical organ and area postrema. The absence of the BBB at these regions means that the parenchyma of the choroid plexuses, pineal gland, pituitary, fornix, hypothalamus and dorsal medulla may be exposed to much higher extracellular levels of xenobiotics than other regions of the brain (Perry & Liebelt, 1961; Ross et al., 1994). The olfactory bulb lies adjacent to capillaries of the olfactory epithelium, separated by only the thin, perforated bone of the cribriform plate. These capillaries lack BBB properties, and blood-borne materials can diffuse into the olfactory bulb (Balin et al., 1986; Ross et al., 1994).

Chemicals that reach the olfactory epithelium via inhalation or topical application may reach the olfactory bulb by diffusing through the olfactory epithelium. However, the many membranes of the olfactory epithelium constitute a considerable physical barrier, and access to the olfactory bulb by airborne chemicals appears to be limited mostly to highly lipophilic materials (Anand-Kumar et al., 1982; Ghantous et al., 1990; Sakane et al., 1991; Lewis et al., 1994).

Xenobiotics reaching the extracellular space in the brain or at extracerebral sites can be taken up by nerve terminals. The vast majority of these xenobiotics will be taken up by fluid-phase endocytosis as part of the normal cell membrane turnover at the nerve terminal. These xenobiotics may be transported retrogradely to the neuronal cell body, where they may be retained in the cytoplasm in lysosomes. For example, this process is thought to contribute significantly to the uptake and retention of heavy metals in the cytoplasm of cell bodies of motor neurons, which project axons into peripheral tissues (Schiønning, 1993; Arvidson, 1994). In contrast, the few materials that are taken up at nerve terminals by adsorptive endocytosis (e.g., lectins) or receptor-mediated endocytosis (e.g., viruses and a few biological toxins) may be transported across several synapses in a process called trans-synaptic transport (Broadwell & Balin, 1985; Shipley, 1985; Spreafico et al., 1985; Baker & Spencer, 1986; Lundh et al., 1988; Astic et al., 1993). Xenobiotics stored in cytoplasmic lysosomes are likely to be retained in the CNS for much longer periods of time than those in the extracellular space.

In the PNS, neuronal cell bodies located in dorsal root ganglia and autonomic ganglia are served primarily by capillaries that lack BBB properties. Nerve fibres projecting centrally and peripherally from these ganglia are provided some protection from large circulating molecules by the presence of connective tissue (perineurium) that separates nerve fascicles and by tight junctions between adjacent endothelial cells of capillaries of the endoneurial lining (Peters et al., 1991). However, the blood–nerve barrier is generally considered to be less efficient than the BBB in limiting access of blood-borne chemicals.

Xenobiotics that reach the extracellular space in the PNS or CNS may contact a variety of cells (e.g., astrocytes, pericytes, microglial cells) that have the capacity to absorb, extrude or metabolize them or to limit their movement in the extracellular space. For example, the foot processes of astrocytes that line cerebral endothelial cells contain a drug-transporting phosphorus-glycoprotein, which intercepts and actively extrudes many blood-borne xenobiotics that manage to reach the CNS extracellular space. However, these cells are in the brain and thus are not, strictly speaking, part of the BBB (Golden & Pardridge, 2000). Moreover, cells performing these functions may sometimes be the target for the toxicant (Aschner, 1996) or enhance the toxicity of the xenobiotic for another cell (Di Monte et al., 1996).

The effectiveness of the BBB, blood–nerve barrier and additional protective cells may be changed by a variety of external factors, including direct chemical damage, infectious disease, elevated body temperature, drugs and changes in serum osmolality. For example, therapeutic drugs handled by the phosphorus-glycoprotein transport system (e.g., vinblastine, loperamide) may temporarily reduce this function via competitive inhibition (for reviews, see Pardridge, 1998). Also, the structural and biochemical features of the BBB have a protracted course during development, and the entry, distribution and exit of materials from the developing nervous system may differ substantially from those in the adult (Neuwelt, 1989; Pardridge, 1998).

3.1.7 Regenerative ability

The nervous system has a combination of special features not found in other organ systems. It is composed of a variety of metabolically active neurons and supporting cell types that interact through a multitude of complex chemical mechanisms. Each cell type has its own functions and vulnerabilities. At the time of puberty, the system is fully developed, and neurogenesis (the birth of new neurons from cell division of precursor cells called neuroblasts) largely ceases. This is in marked and significant contrast to almost all other organs, where cell replacement is continual. Only in specific areas such as the olfactory epithelium does neurogenesis continue. Although recent lines of evidence suggest that "new" neurons can be generated throughout life from neuronal stem cells (Morrison, 1999), there are currently no data to indicate that neurons derived from stem cells in adult life have the capacity to fully integrate into the system and thus provide a source of "replacement neurons" to maintain the normal interactions of the nervous system. While this new evidence demonstrates that the nervous system is even more dynamic than originally thought, the wealth of data on neurodegenerative disease processes and environmentally induced neurodegeneration in the brain suggests that while stem cells may provide a potential source of "new" neurons for the brain, this mechanism is not sufficient to overcome toxic damage.

Unlike many other cell types, neurons do not repair damage to DNA or obviously undergo a continual cycle of programmed cell death and cell replacement. The wealth of data on how the nervous system deals with damage demonstrates a highly complex process of compensation and plasticity of the system (Cotman et al., 1994). CNS neurons are generally unable to be replaced following damage; therefore, the integrated network normally provided is disrupted. As much of the literature has demonstrated, toxic damage to the brain or spinal cord that results in neuronal loss is usually permanent. If such loss is concentrated in one of the CNS's functional subsystems, the outcome could be debilitating; for example, a selective loss of neurons that use acetylcholine as their neurotransmitter may produce a profound disturbance of memory. Similarly, a selective insult concentrated in a subsystem that relies on dopamine as its neurotransmitter may drastically impair motor coordination, as has been demonstrated in Parkinson's disease. Such damage to the nervous system alters the connectivity between the surviving neurons. While neurons do not demonstrate the ability to regenerate in response to injury, they are able to show considerable plasticity both during development and after maturation. This plasticity is often characterized by what has been termed "reactivity synaptogenesis," in that the remaining neurons will demonstrate "sprouting" and formation of new synapses in an attempt to compensate for the damage by providing functional adjustments. Such responsiveness may, in and of itself, have profound consequences for neurological, behavioural and related body functions.

After axons in the peripheral nerves are damaged, they have the ability to regenerate to reach their original target site if the neuronal cell bodies are not damaged. This process is aided by the presence of guide tubes in which the axons can elongate unhindered by scar tissue. This is the basis, for example, of the eventual return of sensation and muscle control in a surgically reattached limb. Neurons in the CNS, most notably in the spinal cord, also have the ability to regenerate interrupted axons; however, they have a much more difficult task in reaching their original targets. This difficulty is thought to be due to the influence of proteins secreted by oligodendrocytes (GrandPre et al.,

2000), which inhibit axonal growth, by the presence of scar tissue formed by proliferating glia and by the possible loss of trophic signals.

3.1.8 Neuroendocrine system

At the base of the brain, several small nuclei in the hypothalamus form the neuroendocrine system, which plays a critical role in the control of the body's endocrine (hormone-secreting) glands (McEwen, 1994). Neuroendocrine dysfunction may occur because of a disturbance in the regulation and/or modulation of neuroendocrine feedback systems. One major indicator of neuroendocrine function is secretion of hormones from the pituitary. Hypothalamic control of anterior pituitary secretions is also involved in a number of important bodily functions. Many types of behaviours (e.g., reproductive behaviours, sexual behaviours in animals) are dependent on the integrity of the hypothalamic–pituitary system, which could represent a potential site of neurotoxicity. Pituitary secretions arise from a number of different cell types in this gland, and neurotoxicants could affect these cells directly or indirectly. Morphological changes in cells mediating neuroendocrine secretions could be associated with adverse effects on the pituitary or hypothalamus and could ultimately affect behaviour and the functioning of the nervous system. Biochemical changes in the hypothalamus may also be used as indicators of potential adverse effects on neuroendocrine function. Finally, the development of the nervous system is intimately associated with the presence of circulating hormones, such as thyroxine (Porterfield, 1994). The nature of the nervous system deficit, which could include cognitive dysfunction, altered neurological development or visual deficits, depends on the severity of the thyroid disturbance and the specific developmental period when exposure to the chemical occurred. In addition, neurobehavioural alterations in response to chemical exposure could be mediated through hormonal interactions. For example, Goldey & Crofton (1998) reported that the hypothyroxinaemia produced by developmental exposure to a mixture of polychlorinated biphenyls (PCBs) was associated with long-term hearing loss. Others (Hany et al., 1999) have reported an increase of sweet preference in association with decreased brain aromatase activity in male offspring of dams treated with a reconstituted PCB mixture. The CNS also regulates the outflow of the endocrine system, which, together with the influence of the autonomic nervous system, can affect immunological function (IPCS, 1986b).

3.1.9   Integrative function of the nervous system

One of the key roles played by the nervous system is to orchestrate the general physiological functions of the body to help maintain homeostasis. To this end, the nervous system and many of the peripheral organ systems are integrated and functionally interdependent. For example, specific neuronal processes are intimately involved in maintaining or modulating respiration, cardiovascular function, body temperature and gastrointestinal function. Because many peripheral organ functions involve neuronal components, changes in such physiological end-points as blood pressure, heart rate, body temperature, respiration, lacrimation or salivation may indirectly reflect possible treatment-related effects on the functional integrity of the nervous system. However, since physiological end-points also depend on the integrity of the related peripheral organ itself, changes in physiological function also may reflect a systemic toxicity involving that organ. Consequently, the neurotoxicological significance of a physiological change must be interpreted within the context of other signs of toxicity. A variety of general physiological procedures can be applied to neurotoxicological problems. These procedures range in scale from simple measurements (e.g., body temperature, respiration, lacrimation, salivation, urination and defecation), which may be included in routine functional observational batteries used for chemical screening, to more involved procedures involving measurements of blood pressure, endocrine responses, cardiac function and gastrointestinal function. The latter would be more appropriate for second-level tests to characterize the scope of chemically related toxicity.

3.2   Toxicological principles

3.2.1   Neurotoxicity

Neurotoxicity can be manifest as a structural or functional adverse response of the nervous system to a chemical, biological or physical agent (Tilson, 1990b; ECETOC, 1992; Ladefoged et al., 1995). It is a function of properties of both the agent and the nervous system itself. It is presumed that neurotoxicity can occur any time during the life cycle, from conception to senescence, and its manifestations can change with age. While responses can often be seen immediately following acute exposure, others may require time for manifestation and are thus often considered to be delayed responses. In either of these cases, the response can show a transient pattern or a more persistent pattern of effect. Effects considered to represent neurotoxicity may or may not be reversible following cessation of exposure. Different responses to the same neurotoxicant can occur, depending upon the dose and timing of exposure. In addition, different agents can produce similar patterns of effects. Expression of neurotoxicity can encompass multiple levels of organization and complexity, including structural, biochemical, physiological and behavioural measurements.

The nervous system is a highly complex and integrated organ. Non-linear dose–response relationships or threshold effects are observed for most agents. It has been hypothesized that the nervous system has a reserve capacity that masks subtle damage. In this case, any exposure that does not overcome this reserve capacity would not reach the threshold, and no impairment would be evident (Tilson & Mitchell, 1983). However, the functional reserve may be depleted over time by a number of factors, including aging, stress or chronic exposure to an environmental insult, and the impairment of functioning and manifestations of toxicity may be delayed in relationship to the exposure. If a number of events occur simultaneously, the response is progressive in nature, or if there is a long latency between exposure and manifestation of toxicity, the identification of a single cause of the functional impairment may not be possible.

Caution must be exercised in labelling a substance neurotoxic. The intended use and effect of the compound, the dose, the exposure scenario and whether or not the compound acts directly or indirectly on the nervous system must be taken into consideration. For example, pharmaceutical agents, vitamins and herbal substances may offer safe and beneficial effects at low concentrations, whereas higher doses may result in neurotoxicity. Therefore, the neurotoxic potential always needs to be considered in terms of the dose relationship.

3.2.2 Structure–activity relationships

Structure–activity relationships (SARs) are widely used to predict toxicological properties of chemicals based on chemical structure. The basis for inference from SARs can be either comparison with structures known to have biological activity or knowledge of structural requirements of a receptor or macromolecular site of action. Although information from SARs can significantly aid in the design of studies, there have been limitations. In neurotoxicology, as in many other areas, there have been relatively few well characterized SARs. Whether this is unique to the nervous system or due to the lack of information on many biological mechanisms underlying neurotoxic actions remains to be determined. However, there are some examples where SARs have been demonstrated and have provided guidance for evaluating additional compounds. Examples include valproate analogues that cause spina bifida (Radatz et al., 1998), hexacarbon diketones that cause peripheral neuropathy (Sanz et al., 1995), organophosphorus compounds predicted to cause organophosphate-induced delayed neurotoxicity (Johnson, 1988) and organic solvents that cause narcosis (Arlien-Søborg, 1992). To date, SARs have been demonstrated only for some specific forms of neurotoxicity; thus, the tacit use of SARs for excluding potential neurotoxicity is not generally acceptable. The SAR approach has been relatively successful in the development of targeted neuropharmacological agents, mostly due to the narrow target defined; even in these cases, however, consideration is required for the potential adverse effects as a result of effects outside of the identified target site. For some homologous groups of chemicals, SARs combined with knowledge of chemical or physical properties have provided information on the risk of acute neurotoxicity or narcotic effects. Data are available for alcohols, ethers, ketones and hydrocarbons (Jeppson, 1975; Hansch & Kim, 1989; Glowa, 1991; Frantik et al., 1994).

Such information is helpful for evaluating potential toxicity when only minimal data are available. The SARs of some chemical classes, such as hexanes, organophosphates, carbamates and pyrethroids, may help predict neurotoxicity or interpret data from neurotoxicological studies. Under certain circumstances (e.g., in the case of new chemicals), this procedure is one of the primary methods used to evaluate the potential for toxicity when few or no empirical toxicity data are available. It should be recognized, however, that effects of chemicals in the same class can vary widely. Moser (1995), for example, reported that the behavioural effects of prototypic cholinesterase-inhibiting pesticides differed qualitatively in a battery of behavioural tests.

3.3   Susceptible populations

Individuals of certain age populations, genetic makeup, health status (e.g., impairment of immune system) and occupations may be at a greater level of risk for neurotoxicity. Fetuses, children and the elderly may be among those in high-risk groups for certain neuro-toxicants (IPCS, 1986a, 1992; Graeter & Mortenson, 1996; Harry & Bruccoleri, 1999). Certain chemical substances may exacerbate existing disorders in certain populations. For example, there is a group of individuals who exhibit a cluster of clinical symptoms that often are referred to as multiple chemical sensitivities. However, there is very little agreement on what the symptoms represent, and a precise definition has not yet been generally endorsed (IPCS, 1999; Kipen & Fiedler, 1999). Data are not available indicating that individuals with this syndrome are more susceptible to neurotoxic agents.

The physiological state, nutritional status and specific nutrient deficiencies (e.g., iron, calcium) can also significantly influence the response to a toxic substance (Ray, 1997).

At any age, pre-existing physical as well as mental disorders of the individual may play a significant role in the manifestation of a toxic response following exposure to a potentially toxic substance. Both types of disorders compromise the system in some way so that the defence mechanisms of the organism are not able to either deal with the toxic substance or repair themselves quickly. In addition to the basic altered biology of individuals with a physical or mental disorder, the combination of therapeutic drugs and toxic substances for those who are under some form of medical intervention may have an interactive effect on the nervous system.

3.3.1   *Developing nervous system*

The development of the mammalian nervous system is a highly complex process, with very specialized morphological and biochemical patterns of organogenesis that continue as a carefully timed multistage process guided by chemical messengers. During embryogenesis, cells multiply at a rapid rate and are relatively undifferentiated. As organogenesis proceeds, cells become more differentiated and migrate to their appropriate location. Other important steps in nervous system development include the formation of synapses, myelination of axons and development of connections between structural components. The temporal and spatial organization of the developmental process is a precise and complex process, with the basic framework laid down in a step-by-step process in which each step is dependent upon the proper completion of the previous one (Rodier, 1990). A relatively minor disturbance resulting in a perturbation of the developmental interactions between selective cells for a limited time may result in a major deleterious outcome.

The developing nervous system appears to be differentially sensitive to some kinds of damage (Cushner, 1981; Pearson & Dietrich, 1985; Annau & Eccles, 1986; Hill & Tennyson, 1986; IPCS, 1986b; Kimmel & Buelke-Sam, 1994). In addition to the critically timed events of CNS development, barriers that will eventually protect much of the adult brain, spinal cord and peripheral nerves are incomplete. The protective mechanisms by which the organism deals with toxic substances, such as the detoxification systems, are not fully developed; thus, adverse effects can result from exposure to some chemicals at lower levels than would be necessary for the average adult (Suzuki, 1980). Exposure to chemicals during development can result in a plethora of effects, ranging from gross structural abnormalities and altered growth to more subtle effects (Spyker, 1975). The qualitative nature of some injuries during development may differ from that of injuries seen in the adult, such as changes in tissue volume, misplaced or misoriented neurons, altered connectivity, and delays in or acceleration of the appearance of functional or structural end-points (Rodier, 1986). In some cases, the results of early injuries may become evident only as the nervous system matures and ages (Riley & Vorhees, 1986; Vorhees, 1987; Rodier, 1990; Kimmel & Buelke-Sam, 1994).

One major factor in determining the type of developmental neurotoxicity manifested is the ontogenetic stage at the time of chemical perturbation (Rodier, 1986). This principle is illustrated by Balduini et al. (1991), who reported that the antimitotic agent methylazoxymethanol produced selective effects on learning and memory in rats depending on the day during gestation on which exposure occurred. If exposure occurred on gestational day 18 or 19, learning deficits were observed, while exposure on earlier days during gestation had no effect. Differential sensitivity of the developing nervous system might be related to the fact that rapidly differentiating cells are highly dependent upon adequate metabolic support. Chemical-induced alterations in brain metabolism could cause different patterns of dysmorphology, depending on the cell types that are differentiating at the time of exposure. It is possible for toxicants to differentially affect specific regions, cell types or cell functions. These damages can be seen at the cellular level and may be due to the targeting of the toxicant by virtue of its chemical properties. The specificity of the damage may be a function of the timing of cells proliferating or differentiating at the time when damaging effects are expressed.

Insult during development can initiate sequences of counter-adaptations and compensatory changes. In all tissues, other than those of the nervous system, cell replacement is an ongoing event; in the nervous system, neurogenesis largely ceases at approximately the time of puberty (although there is evidence of stem cell presence in the mature brain that may offer some ability for limited cell replacement; see section 3.1.7). This loss of neurogenesis limits the nervous system's ability to recover from damage and influences the plasticity of the system. However, in response to injury, the neurons may show considerable responsiveness or plasticity both during development and following maturity. This would permit a limited amount of functional adjustment to occur in compensation. Interpretation of developmental neurotoxicity studies is influenced by the fact that changes observed might well reflect events that are adaptive changes in response to some other injury. However, these adaptive events may compromise the ability of the nervous system to respond to other stressors and so represent an adverse effect in and of themselves.

3.3.2 Aged nervous system

With aging, the level of risk for a number of health-related factors increases; it has been hypothesized that the risk for toxic perturbations to the nervous system also increases with age (Weiss, 1990; IPCS, 1992). It is generally believed that with increasing age comes a decreased ability of the nervous system to respond to adverse events or to compensate for biological, physical or toxic effects. The aging process is thought to result in a reduction of plasticity of the nervous system. Certain pathological lesions (neurofibrillary tangles, abnormal accumulation of certain filamentous proteins) and neuritic plaques are seen more commonly in the CNS of older individuals. It has been postulated that not only might the nervous system become more susceptible to new insults with age, but the effects of previous exposure also may become evident, with a diminished capacity for compensation (Weiss, 1990).

It has been hypothesized that past exposures to environmental chemical agents may contribute to the clinical manifestation of neurodegenerative disorders. Calne et al. (1986) and Steventon et al. (1999) hypothesized that various agents contribute to Alzheimer's disease, Parkinson's disease and amyotrophic lateral sclerosis (ALS, motoneuron disease or Lou Gehrig's disease) by depleting neuronal reserves to an extent that perturbations become observable in the context of the natural aging process. β-N-methylamino-L-alanine, from the seed of the false sago palm (*Cycas circinalis* L.), has been reported to induce a form of ALS associated with dementia in adults (Spencer et al., 1987b). It has been hypothesized that early exposure to the EAA caused neuronal loss, which was added to age-related deficits, leading to early onset of otherwise late neurodegenerative disorders.

3.3.3 Genetic susceptibility

More recent research has suggested that there may be genetic differences between subpopulations that could account for different responses to chemical exposure (Festing, 1991). This has become increasingly evident in the genes associated with neurodegenerative diseases (Steventon et al., 1999). There has yet been no demonstration of a gene–environment interaction with regard to specific chemical-induced neurotoxicity. While there are a limited number of studies examining altered dose–response relationships of specific neurotoxicants in genetically modified animal models, a clear gene–environment association has not been demonstrated. The development and advancement of this experimental approach are dependent upon the establishment of accurate and relevant animal models for the genetically influenced human neurodegenerative diseases.

3.4 Types of effects on the nervous system

Many toxic substances can alter the normal activity of the nervous system. A variety of adverse health effects can be seen, ranging from impairment of movement to disruption of vision and hearing to memory loss and hallucinations (Anger, 1984; IPCS, 1986b; Spencer et al., 2000). Toxic substances can alter both the structure and the function of cells in the nervous system. Structural alterations include changes in the morphology of the cell and its subcellular structures. In some cases, agents produce neuropathic conditions that resemble naturally occurring neurodegenerative disorders in humans (Calne et al., 1986; Ludolph & Spencer, 1995). Cellular alterations can include the accumulation, proliferation or rearrangement of structural elements (e.g., intermediate filaments, microtubules) or organelles (e.g., mitochondria), transport of critical elements and the breakdown of cells. By affecting the biochemistry or physiology of a cell, a toxic substance can alter the internal environment of any neural cell. Intracellular changes can result from oxygen deprivation (anoxia), because neurons require relatively large quantities of oxygen due to their high metabolic rate.

3.4.1 Neurotransmitter function

At the cellular level, a substance might interfere with cellular processes like protein synthesis, leading to a reduced production of neurotransmitters and brain dysfunction (Bondy, 1985). Or a substance might mimic a normal substance in the brain. Organophosphorus compounds, carbamate insecticides and nerve gases act by inhibiting AChE, the enzyme that inactivates the neurotransmitter acetylcholine. Amphetamines stimulate the nervous system by releasing and blocking reuptake of the neurotransmitters norepinephrine and dopamine from nerve cells. Cocaine affects the release and reuptake of norepinephrine, dopamine and serotonin. Amphetamines and cocaine can cause paranoia, hyperactivity, aggression, high blood pressure and abnormal heart rhythms. Opium-related drugs, such as morphine and heroin, act at specific opioid receptors in the brain, producing sedation, euphoria and analgesia. In addition, they can decrease heart rate and breathing patterns and produce nausea and convulsions. Specific effects on neurotransmitters may include perturbation of the system by over-stimulating receptors, blocking transmitter release, inhibiting transmitter degradation and blocking reuptake of neurotransmitter precursors.

3.4.2 Morphological effects

Morphological effects fall into two classes: those that lead to loss of the entire cell (cytotoxicity) and those that lead to loss or rearrangement of structural elements (e.g., axonopathy) without cell death. Both classes of effect may also be seen in naturally occurring neurodegenerative disorders in humans (Calne et al., 1986; Ludolph & Spencer, 1995). All of the cell types in the nervous system may be subject to neurotoxicity, and damage to one cell type (such as the astrocyte) may lead indirectly to damage in others (such as neurons).

An important factor in determining neuronal vulnerability is susceptibility to excitotoxicity. The role of EAA-mediated synaptic activation is critical in normal CNS function. Endogenous EAA-mediated synaptic transmission is essential for many processes, including learning and memory. However, excessive release of endogenous EAAs (such as glutamate) or exposure to exogenous EAAs (such as kainic or domoic acid) can lead to hyperexcitation associated with acute confusion, seizures and weakness. This can lead to neuronal death and memory loss (Choi, 1988). Normally, endogenous EAA release is well controlled, but secondary excitotoxicity is seen in a number of conditions (e.g., epilepsy and vascular damage) that lead to uncontrolled EAA release.

A final common path in many forms of neuronal cytotoxicity is the breakdown of intracellular ionic regulation. A rise in free cytosolic Ca^{2+} results in the release and activation of intracellular enzymes (which break down the cytoskeleton) and the release of stored glutamate, both of which can be cytotoxic (Choi, 1988). The maintenance of ionic gradients imposes a high energy demand on neurons, and impaired oxidative metabolism can thus lead to partial depolarization of resting membrane potential, activation of EAA receptors, influx of Ca^{2+} and Ca^{2+} release from intracellular stores (Riepe et al., 1995).

Cytotoxicity may take the form of necrosis, with cell lysis and consequent reactive changes, or may progress by the more regulated process of programmed cell death or apoptosis. The critical factor determining which form of cell death occurs appears to be mitochondrial energy metabolism; if this is substantially impaired, apoptosis is not possible (Nicotera et al., 1998). Apoptotic death of surplus neurons is seen during normal brain development. Survival of neurons in both the developing and the adult nervous system is dependent on a variety of neurotrophic factors, and deprivation of these can lead to neuronal death. Thus, deprivation of growth factors derived from synaptic input due to the death of one neuron can lead to trans-synaptic death of the next neuron in the chain.

3.4.3 Behaviour

One important aspect of function that may be affected by neurotoxicants is behaviour, which is the product of various sensory, motor and associative functions of the nervous system. Neurotoxic substances can adversely affect sensory or motor functions, disrupt learning and memory processes, or cause detrimental behavioural effects; however, the underlying mechanisms for these effects have yet to be determined. Although changes may be subtle, the assessment of behaviour may serve as a robust means of monitoring the well-being of the organism (Tilson & Cabe, 1978).

3.5 Summary

Advances in neurobiology have improved our understanding of the scientific basis for conducting risk assessments on neurotoxic substances. New information on structure and function of neurons and the cells that support them has led to an understanding that the different expressions of neurotoxicity that are observed have as their bases the different susceptibilities of the various subtypes of cells that make up the nervous system. The cells of the nervous system have special vulnerabilities that are at least partially based on intracellular processes, including (1) intracellular transport of nutrients, structural proteins, organelles and products of catabolism over long distances, (2) the presence of ion channels that make neurons and their processes excitable tissue capable of transmitting signals over long distances in an efficient and reliable manner, and (3) neurotransmission, which allows neurons to communicate with other neurons and other excitable tissue. The important role of the BBB in the CNS and similar structures in the PNS in modulating the access of some chemicals to the brain has become well recognized. Vulnerabilities due to an absence of these barriers in certain parts of the nervous system and the incomplete properties of the barrier are important considerations in assessing the neurotoxicity of some chemicals. Certain specialized cells outside the barrier have a neuroendocrine function that orchestrates important endocrine and metabolic processes. Concepts about the ability of the neurons to replace or regenerate themselves are slowing changing; however, it is generally thought that regenerative capacity in the nervous system is severely constrained and is a limiting factor in achieving full recovery from neurotoxicity under conditions where cell death has occurred.

Assessment of neurotoxicity is complicated by inter-individual and species differences in the response to toxic exposure and by the wide variety of potential effects that chemicals can have on the nervous system. A number of complex testing protocols for adult and developmental neurotoxicity have been developed to identify those structures and functions most likely to be affected by neurotoxic agents. The biological basis for identification of certain populations, including the young, the aged and people with genetic predispositions to certain forms of toxicity, is an important consideration in the risk assessment process for neurotoxicity. Many of the factors that convey susceptibility for neurotoxicity will not differ from those that need to be considered in risk assessments of other target organs, because they involve metabolic processes that are common to many organ systems. In addition to these common vulnerabilities, the long postnatal development process, the complexity of the development process in the nervous system and other factors make the assessment of susceptibility to neurotoxicants more complex. The magnitude of the potential differences in susceptibility of various subpopulations has not been adequately quantified.

4. HUMAN NEUROTOXICITY

4.1 Introduction

During the last 15 years, there has been an increasing number of reports in the literature examining the effects of exposure to neurotoxic agents in humans. The studies are usually case reports or case series involving only a small number of severely affected individuals, while others involve the investigation of larger study groups who may be asymptomatic from a clinical point of view. These studies vary widely, not only with respect to the individuals studied, but also in the methods and study designs they employ, the questions they ask and the inferences that can be made from the information they provide. Despite the many differences in the design of human neurotoxicology studies, they are all, if well conducted, capable of contributing to the risk assessment of particular exposures. However, in order to interpret their findings, it is necessary to understand the inherent advantages and limitations in both the methods and approaches used in different types of studies and the inferences that can be made regarding a causal link between exposure to a particular agent and an adverse health outcome.

For the purpose of discussion, one can think of the development of human neurotoxic disease in the context of a continuum of events. This conceptualization is depicted in Fig. 1.

The initial event on this continuum involves exposure to a neurotoxic substance that can be absorbed in sufficient amounts to produce a biologically effective dose. If the internal level of exposure is sufficiently high, early, reversible biochemical effects may appear, which may provide a means of quantifying exposure or early, non-adverse effects. This assumption of early, readily reversible biochemical effects forms the basis for the search for biochemical markers that can be used in the surveillance of populations at risk for neurotoxic disease. Prolonged exposure at sufficiently high levels may subsequently lead to early health effects that are not of sufficient severity to warrant a clinical diagnosis, but nonetheless are indicative of early signs of neurotoxic effects. The aim of studies examining early nervous system functional effects in exposed populations is also preventative in nature. Such studies typically use measures of health effects that are related or

Exposure → Absorbed dose → Early biological effect →

Altered function → Clinical disease → Disability

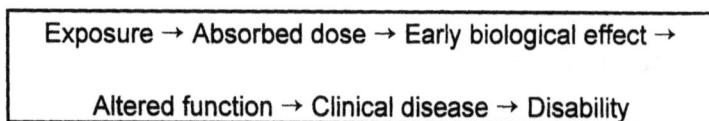

Fig. 1. Continuum between exposure and neurotoxic disease (from Ford et al., 1994).

assumed to be related to disease outcome. They, too, assume that these effects are for the most part reversible in nature and that a reduction of or removal from exposure will prevent progression to frank neurological disease. At the far right of this continuum are studies of individuals who have a history of neurotoxic exposures and present with clinical signs of neurological disease (Ford et al., 1994).

Much of the research in human neurotoxicology over the last decade has centred on the development and validation of techniques to measure functional deficits and the study of neurotoxic effects in adult populations and susceptible populations. The developing nervous system appears to be particularly vulnerable to neurotoxic insult, and a number of studies have correlated environmental exposures with impaired development and nervous system functioning (Needleman, 1990; Jacobson & Jacobson, 1996; Landrigan et al., 2000). Further, it has been suggested that because of a reduced capacity to compensate for impairment, the aging brain may also be particularly vulnerable to neurotoxic insult (Weiss, 2000). The role that genetic factors may play in the metabolism of neurotoxic compounds, consequently altering an individual's susceptibility to neurotoxic disease, is also an area of increasing attention (Feldman & Ratner, 1999).

Different disciplines, including neurology, electrophysiology, psychology, neuroradiology and epidemiology, have contributed to the development of a wide variety of assessment methods and approaches that can be used to evaluate human neurotoxic effects, both clinically and in asymptomatic populations. These techniques and study designs can be used to examine the effects of neurotoxic exposures in working populations as well as persons at risk for neurotoxic illness, including the young and the elderly. In addition, exposure assessment methods derived from industrial hygiene and occupational medicine, methods for measuring and modelling internal levels of exposure derived from the field of toxicokinetics, and the development of biochemical markers of effect are also of importance in our understanding of the relationship between exposure and disease. Some techniques are more appropriate for evaluating individual clinical cases of neurotoxic disease, while others are better suited for population-based studies. The choice of assessment methods depends to some extent on what is known regarding the effects of the compound, the purpose of the evaluation and the feasibility of different methods in different types of studies.

4.2 Methods for assessing human neurotoxicity

4.2.1 Clinical neurological evaluation

The assessment of potential neurotoxicity in individuals begins with a clinical evaluation of an individual patient in order to establish a differential diagnosis of neurotoxic disease and to rule out other possible etiologies. The clinical evaluation of a suspected case of neurotoxicity includes a detailed medical history and a standard clinical neurological examination. Depending on the clinical signs, symptoms or type of exposure, these techniques may be supplemented by other assessment procedures, including clinical neuropsychological evaluation, neurophysiological tests and neuroimaging techniques. Current approaches in the clinical evaluation of neurotoxic disease and descriptions of neurotoxic syndromes associated with exposure to different agents have recently been published (Rosenberg, 1995; Feldman, 1999; Schaumburg, 2000).

The methods and procedures used in the office diagnosis of neurotoxic disease are the same as those used in routine neurological practice. Clinical neurological evaluation begins with an interview and the collection of a medical history. The patient is queried as to past and current medical conditions and current medications, the health of family members, use of alcohol and recreational drugs, and hobbies. Detailed information is also obtained regarding the agent to which the patient was exposed, occupational duties, the route and duration of exposure and whether co-workers are also affected. This information is of paramount importance, as it may be the only information available to the clinician at intake regarding the possible role of exposure in the etiology of the patient's disorder. Information obtained from the medical and occupational history can often serve as a guide for focusing on specific end-points during the neurological examination.

The neurological examination begins with a brief assessment of mental status, including level of consciousness, orientation, disorders of speech (i.e., dysphasia, dysarthria, dysphonia), concentration, memory, mood and affect. Cranial nerve function is also examined. Motor system evaluation includes inspection for muscle atrophy, unusual movements, tremor and gait abnormalities. In addition, an analysis of coordination, muscle tone and resistance to passive stretch and an assessment of strength of individual muscles are conducted. Assessment of cutaneous sensory function, including pain, position, vibration, light touch and temperature, is also carried out. Finally, tendon reflexes and the plantar responses to cutaneous stimulation are also determined (Bradley et al., 1996).

Depending on the presentation of signs and symptoms and the nature of the exposure, more specialized evaluations may also be indicated. In addition, an assessment of exposure may also be carried out (Chern et al., 1995). A description of these methods both in the evaluation of clinical cases and in epidemiological studies of exposed populations is presented below.

4.2.2 *Neuropsychological and neurobehavioural testing*

4.2.2.1 *Individual neuropsychological assessment*

In addition to the neurological examination, neuropsychological testing is often carried out in the clinical evaluation of neurotoxicity, especially in those cases where there is an indication of cognitive or affective changes (Feldman, 1999; Schaumburg, 2000). Similar to the neurological examination, neuropsychological testing also helps in ruling out other etiologies as well as establishing the extent of psychological impairment.

Clinical evaluation includes a structured interview and formal psychological testing (White et al., 1992). Because toxic exposures may produce neuropsychiatric disorders, tests of emotional functioning are also carried out (Bolla & Roca, 1994). In addition, tests to assess the under- or overreporting of symptoms (i.e., malingering or dissimulation) may also be administered. Specific methods for the detection of malingering in neuropsychological or psychiatric test settings or questionnaire-based information collection are available (Nies & Sweet, 1994). Although different clinical neuropsychologists may use somewhat different tests for evaluating neurotoxicity (e.g., Lezak, 1983; Hartman, 1988; White et al., 1992; Agnew & Masten, 1994), the choice of tests is, in general, aimed at assessing a wide range of functions, including different aspects of verbal function, visuospatial ability, memory, attention, cognitive tracking and flexibility, and psychomotor abilities. As the purpose of the clinical evaluation is the differential diagnosis of the patient's condition, and as the patient may possibly have a neurological condition unrelated to toxic exposure, clinical testing cannot be limited to the administration of one or two "sensitive" tests administered in a "blind" fashion. Instead, it requires the sampling of a comprehensive array of cognitive, affective and neurobehavioural functions. This information must be interpreted in the context of the patient's premorbid intellectual level of functioning and interpersonal adjustment. Examples of tests from a clinical neuropsychological battery are presented in Table 2.

The Wechsler Adult Intelligence Scale–Revised (WAIS-R) is one of the most widely used instruments for estimating overall intellectual functioning or intelligence quotient (IQ). Although overall IQ measures have been shown to be affected by lead exposure in children (Needleman et al., 1979a,b, 1990), adult IQ estimates computed from the Wechsler scales or other measures have not, in general, been found to be particularly sensitive to neurotoxic exposure. Estimates of overall intellectual functioning, however, are necessary in order to adequately interpret deficits on particular tests in the context of the patient's general level of intellectual functioning. Further, several WAIS-R subtests (e.g., Digit Symbol, Similarities and Digit Span) appear to be sensitive to neurotoxic exposures. In contrast, the WAIS-R subtests Information and Vocabulary are typically used with other neuropsychological tests, e.g., Wide-range Achievement Test and the Peabody Picture Vocabulary Test, as "hold" tests, or tests that can be used to help infer premorbid levels of functioning.

Clinical neuropsychological testing is carried out on a one-to-one basis by a trained examiner, and results must be interpreted by an experienced clinical neuropsychologist. Often, five or more hours are

Table 2. Examples of tests in a clinical neuropsychological battery[a]

Domain/tests	Description/comments
General intellect	
Wechsler Adult Intelligence Scale–Revised (WAIS-R)	Full-scale IQ, Verbal IQ and Performance IQ constitute measures of general level of cognitive ability compared with population norms; some subtests can serve as "hold" tests
Peabody Picture Vocabulary Test	Measure of verbal intelligence in adults
Wide-range Achievement Test	Measures academic skills in arithmetic, spelling, reading; used to estimate premorbid ability patterns in adults
Attention and executive function	
Digit Span Subtest (WAIS-R)	Immediate recall of digits forwards and backwards; measures simple attention and tracking
Trail Making Test	Connect-a-dot task; measures attention, sequencing, scanning
Continuous Performance Test	Automated test of attention
Paced Auditory Serial Addition	Serial calculation tests; sensitive measure of attention/tracking
Wisconsin Card Sorting Test	Requires inference of decision-making rules; assesses mental flexibility
Verbal ability and language	
Information Subtest (WAIS-R)	Recall of information usually learned in school; robust estimate of native ability in adults
Vocabulary Subtest (WAIS-R)	Fairly robust estimate of verbal intelligence in adults
Similarities Subtest (WAIS-R)	Calls for inference of similarities between nominative words; assesses verbal reasoning
Boston Naming Test	Naming of objects from line drawings; sensitive to aphasia
Visuospatial and visuomotor	
Digit Symbol Subtest (WAIS-R)	Requires matching symbols to digits; assesses perceptual coding and motor speed
Rey-Osterreith Complex Figure	"Copy condition" assesses visuospatial planning and construction
Santa Ana Form Board	Measures motor speed and coordination
Finger Tapping Test	Electronic or mechanical counting of finger tapping speed

Table 2 (Contd).

Domain/tests	Description/comments
Memory	
Wechsler Memory Scale–Revised	Assesses learning and retention of verbal and visual material
California Verbal Learning Test	Provides multiple measures of new verbal learning, recall, recognition memory, use of strategies, inference
Rey-Osterreith Complex Figure	Recall condition assesses memory for complex visual information
Mood and personality	
Profile of Mood States (POMS)	Multiple scales of severity ratings of affective symptoms; sensitive to mood disturbance and affective changes
Minnesota Multiphasic Personality Inventory–Revised (MMPI-R)	Personality inventory; provides description of current personality function; some scales sensitive to toxic exposures

ª From White & Proctor (1995).

required to complete a clinical neuropsychological evaluation. Such an evaluation is obviously quite extensive, in terms of both time and scope. In contrast, experimental and epidemiological studies typically require the use of tests that can be administered in a much shorter period of time than that needed for a full clinical evaluation, but are equally or more sensitive in detecting neurotoxic effects. Moreover, the use of neurobehavioural testing methods in experimental and epidemiological study designs requires the use of blind testing procedures, particularly if techniques are not automated. Further, statistical analyses are used in order to judge the evidence for neurotoxic effects. Several approaches to the use of neurobehavioural methods in these types of studies are presented below.

!.2.2.2   Cognitive testing batteries

One approach to evaluating changes in neurobehavioural functioning in studies of exposed populations involves a shortened battery of clinical neuropsychological tests that focus on those effects most commonly seen in CNS toxic disorders. Such an approach was taken in one of the first studies reporting neurobehavioural changes in carbon disulfide-exposed workers conducted at the Finnish Institute of Occupational Health by Hänninen (1971). Subsequently, the use of selected neuropsychological tests to evaluate exposed populations was adopted by a number of investigators (Baker et al., 1984; Cherry et al., 1984; Ryan et al., 1987; Hänninen, 1990b; Bowler et al., 1991).

In an attempt to standardize test methods in the field of human neurotoxicology, a Neurobehavioral Core Test Battery (NCTB) (Table 3) was published by WHO for use, on an international scale, in epidemiological studies (Johnson et al., 1987). For the most part, the battery is composed of easy-to-administer paper-and-pencil tests also used in clinical assessments, with the exception of the Santa Ana Form Board Test and the Simple Reaction Time Test.

Table 3. WHO Neurobehavioural Core Test Battery (NCTB)[a]

Domain	Test
Perceptual coding	Digit Symbol (WAIS-R)
Attention and short-term memory	Simple Reaction Time Digit Span (WAIS-R) Benton Visual Recognition
Psychomotor performance	Aiming Motor Santa Ana Form Board
Mood and affect	Profile of Mood States (POMS) Questionnaire

[a] Adapted from Anger (1990).

In general, the NCTB is relatively inexpensive and easy to administer. It has been successfully used in a variety of different cultures, although difficulties with its use in some developing countries have been noted. Further, the NCTB has a large base of control data (Anger et al., 1993) and consists of tests that have most consistently identified neurotoxic effects in occupational settings (Anger et al., 2000). Its major disadvantage is that it requires an examiner who can test only one person at a time, and the paper-and-pencil nature of the tests requires a considerable amount of interaction between the examiner and the subject, which could conceivably influence test results.

With the advent of low-cost computer technology, it is possible to use automated methods for administering tests and recording the person's response accurately and objectively. At present, a number of different automated test batteries have been developed (Hartman, 1995; Iregren, 1998). Examples of some of these batteries are listed in

Table 4. In some cases (e.g., the Neurobehavioural Evaluation System, or NES), tests in the battery were meant to provide an automated version of paper-and-pencil neuropsychological tests, while in others (e.g., Swedish Performance Evaluation System, or SPES), tests were designed on the basis of theoretical considerations derived from experimental psychology. Test procedures based on operant methods have also been described (Paule et al., 1990).

Table 4. Some automated test batteries used in neurotoxicology research[a]

System name	Number of tests	Number of rating scales	Reference
Behavioural Assessment & Research System	4	0	Anger et al. (1994)
Cognitive Function Scanner	8	0	Laursen (1990)
Information Processing & Performance Test Battery	8	0	Williamson (1990)
Milan Automated Neurobehavioural System	7	0	Cassito et al. (1989)
Microtox System	17	0	Eckerman et al. (1985)
Neurobehavioural Evaluation System (NES)	17	1	Baker et al. (1985)
Swedish Performance Evaluation System (SPES)	18	5	Gamberale et al. (1990)

[a] Adapted from Iregren (1998).

An important advantage of computerized tests is that computers can consistently present test materials in a standardized manner and cannot inadvertently cue or prompt the subject. Further, the automatic recording of responses and response latencies can also be accurately performed, and complex scoring systems can be incorporated into the test program. Thus, because an automated approach allows for the exact timing of stimulus presentation and speed of response, quite subtle effects on the accuracy, speed and patterning of responding can be measured. The major drawback of automated testing, at least at present, is the limited stimulus material that can be presented and the limited types of responses that can be recorded. Most computerized tests rely almost exclusively on the visual presentation of material, and the type of response is restricted to the handling of keyboards, joysticks and push buttons. In contrast, in examiner-administered tests derived from clinical neuropsychology, the mode of stimulus presentation may be visual or verbal in nature. Further, the response modality is also quite varied for different clinical test instruments. For some examiner-administered tests, a verbal response is required, while for others, the manipulation of test materials is called for. Thus, at this time, the range of functions that can be assessed by automated tests is less than that afforded by examiner-administered neuropsychological test instruments. For example, different aspects of fine and gross motor abilities, expressive language, constructional disorders and astereognosis cannot be evaluated using computerized testing techniques.

Although some computerized and hand-administered tests appear to test similar functions (and in some cases have similar names, e.g., the Digit Symbol Subtest in the WHO NCTB and the Symbol Digit Substitution Test in the NES), computerized and non-computerized tests differ along a number of dimensions, including the size, duration and presentation of stimuli, number of trials, response modality and scoring procedures. In studies designed to compare performance on computerized and hand-administered tests, only modest to weak positive correlations have been found (Bowler et al., 1990). Thus, results obtained with seemingly similar computerized and non-computerized tests are not directly comparable, despite the fact that both versions of a particular test may have been designed to assess the same psychological domain.

Recently, a test battery combining both hand-administered and computerized tests, the Adult Environmental Neurobehavioral Test Battery (AENTB), has been proposed by the Agency for Toxic Substances and Disease Registry in the USA. The AENTB is intended for use in studies examining the effects of neurotoxic exposures in persons located in the vicinity of hazardous waste sites (Anger et al., 1994). This battery consists of tests from the WHO-recommended NCTB, computerized tests from the NES and additional behavioural neurophysiological tests of sensory and motor function not in those batteries (Amler et al., 1995).

Considerable progress has been made over the last two decades in examining the psychometric properties of different examiner-administered and computerized test batteries and in validating their use for examining the effects of neurotoxic exposures in exposed populations.

For the WHO-recommended NCTB, normative data for tests in this battery have been collected on an international scale from over 2300 non-exposed control subjects in 10 European countries, North and Central America, and Asia for five age ranges from 16 to 65 years (Anger et al., 1993). Factor analysis studies (Hooisma et al., 1990) have indicated that the NCTB tests load on five factors, including perceptual speed, immediate memory, reaction time, motor coordination and speed, and learning and memory. Although the NCTB is not always administered as a battery *per se*, tests in the battery have often been used in combination with other psychological test instruments for evaluating the effects of exposure to a wide range of human neurotoxicants (for review, see Johnson et al., 1987; White et al., 1992). Some examples of recent studies using these NCTB tests include the examination of the effects of low-level exposure to metals (Chia et al., 1997), solvents (Escalona et al., 1995; Mergler et al., 1996) and pesticides (London et al., 1997). Studies using different WHO NCTB tests, either alone or in combination with other tests, have indicated that these tests are sensitive in detecting the neurotoxic effects of a wide range of different compounds. Moreover, these tests can be applied in different cultures, although difficulties in testing persons with no or little education have been reported (Anger et al., 1993).

Of the automated test batteries currently in use, the NES, developed in the early 1980s, is the most widely used computerized test system (US OTA, 1990). Similar to the NCTB tests, the NES battery has been extensively validated in the neurotoxicology literature, with over 40 publications describing its use in cross-sectional and experimental exposure studies (Letz, 1991, 1993; Anger et al., 1994, 2000). Recently, a number of NES subtests have been successfully applied to the study of environmental pollutants in young school-aged children (Altmann et al., 1997). The SPES, developed in Sweden, has also been extensively validated and used in experimental laboratory studies and cross-sectional studies of workers exposed to solvents, aluminium, manganese and physical factors (Gamberale et al., 1990; Iregren, 1998). Further, both the NES and SPES have been translated into a variety of different languages, which helps improve the comparability of the results of studies conducted in different countries using these automated techniques.

A common characteristic of psychological test instruments is that they are exquisitely sensitive to a host of subject variables that should

Table 5. Subject variables that may potentially confound or modify study outcome in neurobehavioural studies[a]

Stable factors	Situational factors
■ age of subject	■ alcohol (recent use)
■ educational level	■ caffeine (recent use)
■ sex	■ nicotine (recent use)
■ socioeconomic group or occupation	■ medicines or drugs (recent use)
■ first language	■ paints, glues or pesticides (recent use)
■ preferred hand	
■ computer experience (automated tests only)	■ near visual acuity
	■ upper body injury restricting movement
■ caffeine (habitual use)	■ recent cold or flu
■ alcohol (habitual use)	■ stress
■ nicotine (habitual use)	■ arousal (and fatigue), sleep last night
■ medicines or drugs (habitual use)	
■ paints, glues or pesticides (habitual use)	■ screen luminance (automated tests only)
■ diabetes	■ time of day
■ epilepsy	■ time of year
■ other nervous system disease	
■ head injury causing unconsciousness > 1 h	
■ alcohol or drug addiction	
■ level of physical activity at work	

[a] Adapted from Stephens & Barker (1998).

be considered in the design and interpretation of neurotoxicity studies (Stephens & Barker, 1998). A list of factors that may potentially confound or modify the outcome of cross-sectional neurobehavioural studies is presented in Table 5. In systematic studies examining the psychometric properties of the NCTB and NES, for example, different tests have been shown to be sensitive to a variety of factors, including age, educational level, cultural group and gender, depending on the test (Anger et al., 1997). Visual acuity may also be important in the performance of automated tests (Hudnell et al., 1996). Reports in the literature indicate that severe problems with the interpretation of neuropsychological studies can result when critical confounding factors are not controlled for (Gade et al., 1988). Findings such as these have led to the publication of criteria for the evaluation of human neurobehavioural studies of neurotoxicity by the EC (1996) to help risk assessors judge the quality of human studies.

Psychiatric and symptom questionnaires

Changes in affect are some of the most dramatic effects of severe neurotoxic exposures (Bolla & Roca, 1994). Psychotic symptoms, including delusions, hallucinations and paranoia, have been noted in mercury, arsenic and manganese poisoning cases (White & Proctor, 1995), and suicidal depression resulting from poisoning with carbon disulfide has been well known for over a century (Mikkelsen, 1995). Less severe effects (e.g., changes in mood and energy levels) have also been reported in exposed populations and, in some cases, may be the earliest indication of neurotoxic exposure (IPCS, 1986b). As a result, questionnaires and symptom ratings are also typically included both in the assessment of individual neurotoxicity cases and in epidemiological studies of exposed populations.

In the clinic, the revised edition of the Minnesota Multiphasic Personality Inventory (MMPI-R), which contains over 500 items requiring a yes/no response, can be used to assess personality and psychological functioning in individual patients (Bolla & Roca, 1994; White & Proctor, 1995). Because of its length and the nature of some of the questions, however, the MMPI is poorly suited for cross-sectional studies of exposed populations. One clinical test instrument that has been more widely used in cross-sectional studies is the Profile of Mood States Questionnaire (POMS), which is a 65-item rating scale of mood state. Modified versions of the POMS have been incorporated into the NCTB and NES test batteries for use in cross-sectional studies.

In addition, a number of questionnaires and rating scales have been specifically developed to obtain information in a standardized manner regarding subjective complaints associated with neurotoxic exposure (e.g., Hänninen, 1971; Hogstedt et al., 1984; Hooisma et al., 1994; Chouaniere et al., 1997). For example, the Q16 questionnaire consists of 16 yes/no questions designed to elicit information regarding symptoms of the early effects of neurotoxic exposures in working populations (Hogstedt et al., 1984). Validation studies of the Q16 have examined its test–retest reliability, its sensitivity in discriminating exposed and non-exposed populations, and its ability to predict other outcome measures (Lundberg et al., 1997; Smargiassi et al., 1998). The Neurotoxic Symptom Checklist-60 (NSC-60) consists of 53 questions designed to elicit information regarding mood and affect, absent-mindedness and memory problems, sensory and motor disturbances, chest problems, equilibrium disturbances, somatic problems, fatigue and sleep disturbances, as well as 7 personality items (Hooisma et al., 1994). The NSC-60 is being used in cross-sectional studies of exposed workers (Ruijten et al., 1994; Viaene et al., 2000), in the occupational health care setting for the surveillance of workers exposed to neurotoxic compounds, and in the evaluation of suspected neurotoxicity cases (van der Laan et al., 1995). In Germany, an analogue rating scale has been developed, and the consistency of ratings from this instrument in experimental exposure studies and its ability to discriminate exposed and non-exposed populations have been evaluated (Kieswetter et al., 1997; Seeber et al., 1997).

Although the reporting of subjective symptoms may be a valid, early indicator of neurotoxicity, self-report data are notable for the different types of reporting bias that may influence them. Respondents may either consciously or unknowingly bias the answer to fit what they believe to be the examiner's expectations, and the recall of details of objective events or subjective states may alter with the passage of time. Further, because characteristics such as gender and affiliation of the tester may also affect responding, these variables need to be controlled for in cross-sectional studies.

In group studies, biases in self-report data can be reduced by making the questionnaire anonymous or highly confidential. Objective data can sometimes be obtained to help validate self-reports. The objective measurement of behaviour or biological samples, for example, may help corroborate self-report data. Further, many structured clinical interviews and self-report assessment instruments include some mechanisms for detecting self-report bias, either by looking for endorsement of improbable behaviours or by examining the consistency of information gathered in several ways or from several sources. Concordance between subjective symptoms, objective measures and documented levels of exposure increases the judged validity of self-reports.

1.2.2.4 Behavioural neurophysiological tests

Because sensory and motor changes have often been associated with exposure to particular chemicals, both the neurological examination and symptom questionnaires typically include items designed to obtain information regarding sensory and motor disturbances. In recent years, however, several behavioural methodologies have been used to provide quantitative measures of different aspects of visual, somato-sensory and olfactory function (Mergler, 1995). In addition, quantitative measures have been developed to examine the effects of chemicals on postural balance and tremor (Araki et al., 1997). Typically, these techniques are not used in the clinical evaluation of individual patients. Rather, they have been developed for the purpose of monitoring and health surveillance in field studies of exposed workers. Behavioural neurophysiological tests constitute part of the AENTB described above (Anger et al., 1994; Amler et al., 1995). Although neurotoxic exposures have been associated with effects on different sensory modalities, including hearing (e.g., Morata & Dunn, 1994), most of the work in the area of behavioural neurophysiological testing has concentrated on colour vision, contrast sensitivity, vibration sensitivity and olfactory discrimination.

With respect to colour vision, colour arrangement tests, such as the Lanthony D-15 desaturated (LD15-D) hue panel and the Farns-worth-Munsell 100 (FM-100) hue panel, have been shown to be sensitive to neurotoxin-induced colour vision loss (Mergler, 1995). In both tests, the subject is required to arrange different coloured caps in order of colour similarity. These tests can distinguish between congenital colour vision loss and acquired colour vision loss due to neurotoxic exposure. Following initial reports of colour vision loss in *n*-hexane-exposed workers (Raitta et al., 1978), colour arrangement tests have been used to examine colour vision changes in workers exposed to a number of different solvents, including carbon disulfide (Ruijten et al., 1990), styrene (Gobba et al., 1991), toluene (Zavalić et al., 1998) and mixed organic solvents (Broadwell et al., 1995).

In addition to tests of colour vision, tests of visual contrast sensitivity are also available for examining changes in visual acuity. Contrast sensitivity threshold testing involves the presentation of sinusoidal gratings at different spatial frequencies in order of decreasing contrast. Subjects are required to indicate the direction of the gratings with three different presentations being used to ascertain the threshold. Contrast sensitivity patterns differing in spatial frequencies appear to be differentially sensitive to disturbances in different parts of the visual system. Whereas a loss of acuity at high spatial frequencies is generally associated with optical changes, loss of acuity at intermediate and low spatial frequencies has been associated with changes at the neural level.

Recent studies suggest that changes in contrast sensitivity at intermediate frequencies may also be sensitive to solvent effects (Broadwell et al., 1995).

With respect to the somatosensory system, behavioural techniques for assessing changes in vibration sensitivity using psychophysical procedures have also been described (Arezzo et al., 1983; Muijser et al., 1986; Gerr & Letz, 1988). The basic design of the equipment includes a vibrating shaft that protrudes through a hole in a metal base plate. Stimuli of varying amplitude are then presented to the subject. Two different psychophysical procedures have been utilized, the forced choice method and the method of limits. Comparative studies of the two procedures indicate that the method of limits appears to be a more reliable and efficient procedure (Gerr & Letz, 1988). One of the difficulties in the use of vibration sensitivity testing is the lack of standardized equipment and testing methods. Important differences in the physical characteristics of the different measuring devices exist, with some instruments unable to control for the influence of pressure exerted by the subject on stimulus amplitude of the vibrating shaft. In addition, vibration sensitivity threshold is affected by a number of other factors (e.g., age, height, gender, illness) unrelated to exposure that should be controlled for in the conduct of studies using this approach (Gerr et al., 1990; Gerr & Letz, 1993).

In addition to behavioural tests to evaluate visual and somatosensory function, tests to examine odour identification and olfactory perception threshold have also been described (Mergler, 1995). The most commonly used odour identification kit is the University of Pennsylvania smell identification kit, which includes four booklets of microencapsulated odorants. The odorant is released by scratching a pencil over the odorant strip, and the subject's task is to identify the odour by choosing one of four answers. To evaluate odour threshold perception, serial solutions of a particular substance are presented to the subject, and the subject is required to indicate which of two bottles contains the odorant using a forced choice procedure.

Finally, quantitative methods for examining postural sway are also being used in epidemiological and laboratory investigations of effects of pesticides and solvents and might be useful for assessing therapeutic drug-induced movement disorders as well. Measurement of postural stability requires a computer, special software, monitor and a force transduction platform on which the subjects must stand (Dick et al., 1990; Araki et al., 1997). Mechanical and capacitive field methods for assessing the amplitude and frequency of tremor also are seeing more frequent use (Newland, 1997).

4.2.3 Electrophysiological tests

Similar to behavioural tests, electrophysiological tests of PNS and CNS function may be used to augment the neurological examination. Although these tests are not in themselves diagnostic of neurotoxicity, they can be used to help detect and characterize dysfunction. Electrophysiological methods are generally used to diagnose individual patients but could be applied to the study of exposed populations, particularly exposed workers. One advantage of electrophysiological tests is that many techniques are directly applicable to animal studies, making possible direct cross-species comparisons.

Routine electrophysiological evaluations, including nerve conduction velocity (NCV) testing and needle electromyography (EMG), are widely used quantitative methods for examining peripheral nerve and muscle function in clinical evaluation (Jabre, 1995; Schaumburg, 2000). In contrast to EMG recordings, NCV studies can be conducted with surface electrodes, making NCV techniques quite suitable for epidemiological studies of exposed populations (Araki et al., 1997; Seppäläinen, 1998). NCV measurements are based on the fact that when a nerve is electrically stimulated, an electrical response can be recorded, and the time relationship between the stimulus and response can be described. For motor conduction velocity (MCV) studies, the indirect motor action potential can be obtained by stimulating the motor nerve using a supramaximal intensity stimulus and recording from an electrode located on the muscle that it innervates. Responses can be characterized in terms of latency, amplitude, duration, area and waveform. Sensory nerve action potentials (NAPs) are obtained by stimulating and recording from a nerve or one of its branches. The NAP is also characterized by its amplitude, duration and waveform. Changes in the amplitude of the sensory NAP are the most sensitive measures of axonal dysfunction in sensory nerves. Because NCV studies can discriminate the proximal versus distal nature of axonal dysfunction, they are particularly important for the determination of neurotoxic disease (Schaumburg, 2000).

In addition to routine methods for evaluating peripheral nerve function, quantitative techniques have also been recently developed for detecting abnormalities at an earlier stage or for use when the results of routine conduction velocity studies are normal (Jabre, 1995; Araki et al., 1997). These techniques include the mean related values technique and the distribution of conduction velocities technique. The mean related values technique is the statistical analysis of an individual's values in terms of their Gaussian or non-Gaussian distribution compared with normal reference values. The advantages of this approach are an increase in sensitivity, the ability to express all data using a single unit (i.e., the standard deviation) and the ability to assess the degree of severity (Jabre, 1995). With the distribution of conduction velocities technique (Araki et al., 1997), an estimate of the conduction velocities of medium and smaller fibres, as well as those of the largest and fastest fibres, is possible. The information obtained with this methodology may help in differentiating toxin-induced peripheral neuropathies from other neurological diseases of the PNS (Araki et al., 1997).

Electrophysiological techniques for evaluating CNS dysfunction include electroencephalography (EEG) and different types of evoked potentials (EPs). The EEG is the summed electrical activity of neurons and is measured non-invasively with scalp electrodes. In the clinic, EEG is useful primarily in evaluating and classifying seizure disorders. EEG was the earliest electrophysiological test to be applied in industrial medicine and may be helpful in monitoring acute poisoning cases (Seppäläinen, 1988). However, the pattern of abnormality is rarely associated with a specific compound (Schaumburg, 2000), thus limiting the use of the EEG for diagnosing neurotoxic disease. EEG has been used in cross-sectional studies of exposed populations, particularly workers exposed to organic solvents, with variable findings. These studies have been recently reviewed (Seppäläinen, 1998).

With the development of computer technology, it is now possible to record and store the EEG digitally, so that the information can be easily accessed and reproduced for display and analysis. Digital EEG is directly analogous to paper EEG recordings and is a significant improvement of this technology.

The availability of digitized EEG data has also led to the development of a host of quantitative EEG (qEEG) methodologies, whereby the digital EEG is mathematically processed in order to extract particular features for analysis and comparison (Nuwer, 1997). Different types of qEEG include signal analysis, such as automated event detection and frequency analysis; topographic displays or "brain mapping"; and statistical analysis methods designed to compare an individual on some parameter with normative values or to compare different subgroups of patients for the purpose of diagnostic discriminant analysis.

Despite their potential advantages, the clinical usefulness of qEEG techniques is at present quite limited, although they may have substantial usefulness for future applications. As pointed out in a recent review (Nuwer, 1997), techniques used for qEEGs vary widely between laboratories, making comparison of results difficult. In addition, besides being subject to traditional EEG artefacts, qEEG data may produce new artefacts caused by the data-processing algorithms that are difficult to detect and interpret. Moreover, important abnormal activity may be missed as well. For these and other reasons, the use of qEEG for differential diagnosis in the clinic has been discouraged at this time (Nuwer, 1997; Schaumburg, 2000). Despite these limitations, however, some very interesting studies of solvent and pesticide exposure (e.g., Jonkman et al., 1992), drug abuse (e.g., Struve et al., 1994) and psychiatric disorders (e.g., Prichep & John, 1992) have been reported.

In contrast to EEG, EPs are electrical cortical responses elicited by specific stimulation of specific sensory pathways or complex endogenous events (Araki & Murata, 1993; Otto & Hudnell, 1993; Otis & Handler, 1995). Sensory evoked potentials (SEPs) are produced by peripheral sensory stimuli (e.g., auditory, visual, somatosensory or chemical), are time-locked to the stimulus and occur with consistent, reproducible waveforms and latencies. In the clinic, the most commonly used EPs are the visual evoked potential (VEP), the brainstem auditory evoked potential (BAEP) and the somatosensory evoked potential (SSEP). Chemosensory evoked potentials (CSEPs) have been used in research studies but are rarely used in clinical evaluations. When properly performed and interpreted, SEPs can be used to evaluate the integrity of a sensory system from the receptor in the periphery to the cerebral cortex. Event-related potentials (ERPs) are another category of EPs. These potentials (e.g., P300, cognitive evoked potentials) are produced by the processing of complex information and may be useful in evaluating cognitive processes. Similar to qEEG techniques, some very interesting research studies have been conducted with ERPs (e.g., Steinhauer et al., 1997). However, ERPs have no known clinical utility at this time (Schaumburg, 2000).

SEP testing has been used in a number of neurotoxicology studies to examine the neurotoxic effects of solvents, metals and pesticides in exposed populations, as well as in experimental exposure studies (Otis & Handler, 1995; Seppäläinen, 1998). Pattern-shift VEPs have been found to be sensitive to several organic solvents, including *n*-hexane (e.g., Chang, 1987), and changes in BAEPs of lead-exposed workers have also been reported (e.g., Discalzi et al., 1993).

Further, dose–response functions have been found with EP methods. For example, a curvilinear relationship was found between BAEP and blood lead concentrations in children (Otto & Hudnell, 1990), and a biphasic function was reported for VEP latency and tetrachloroethylene exposure concentration in a laboratory study (Altmann et al., 1991). In the latter study, the direction of the response was jointly dependent on dose and stimulus parameters. In addition, changes over time in the effect of the solvent on VEP were dose and stimulus parameter dependent.

Two important methodological considerations are illustrated by BAEP and VEP data. One is that low concentrations of some chemical agents may produce effects (shorter latencies in these examples) that could be interpreted as facilitation rather than impairment. However, one should bear in mind that changes in neuronal latencies in either direction could be a result of a neurotoxic process. The second consideration is that the detection of neurotoxic effects is dependent on dose–time–testing parameter interactions. A thorough understanding of the effects of testing parameters on the dose–response relationship and the time course of chemical effects is necessary for adequately interpreting the results of neurotoxicity studies.

Recent developments in quantitative neurophysiological methods provide promising research tools for the evaluation of neurotoxicity in humans. Techniques such as peripheral nerve testing and SEPs have been used extensively in the clinic for diagnostic purposes and have been used successfully to provide objective data of peripheral nerve and sensory abnormalities in exposed populations. Other methods, such as qEEG, the analysis of the P300 waveform and ERPs, have shown differences at the group level. However, further research aimed at standardizing techniques, validating different methodologies and examining the effects of different exposures is necessary before such methods can be accepted as diagnostic instruments.

4.2.4 Neuroimaging techniques

Over the last 20 years, a number of image-producing technologies, such as computerized axial tomography (CAT), magnetic resonance imaging (MRI), positron emission tomography (PET) and single photon emission computerized tomography (SPECT), have been developed for use in the diagnosis of neurological disease. CAT and MRI produce images of the brain, and PET and SPECT supply functional or biochemical information that cannot be obtained with other methods in a non-invasive manner. Neuroimaging techniques provide an invaluable measure of local brain function and dysfunction, which can be integrated with neurobehavioural measures for studying brain–behaviour relationships at the human level.

Neuroimaging methods have proven extremely useful in the diagnosis of certain neurological diseases and are being increasingly used in neurotoxicity studies (see Prockop, 1995; Sullivan et al., 1998; Trieberg, 1998). They have been used successfully to document brain pathology in a number of different types of acute neurotoxic poisoning cases as well as patients suspected of chronic neurotoxicity. Examples include studies on carbon monoxide (Gale et al., 1999; Prockop & Naidu, 1999), solvents (White et al., 1993; Heuser & Mena, 1994; Thuomas et al., 1996; Hageman et al., 1999), solvent abuse (Caldemeyer et al., 1996; Yamanouchi et al., 1998), heavy metals (Nelson et al., 1993), pesticides (Callender et al., 1994; Heuser & Mena, 1994) and drug abuse (Aasly, 1993).

The reports cited above as well as others in the literature are typically based on small numbers of patients, and the exposures are not well characterized and may involve co-exposure of the patients to other, unidentified neurotoxicants. This is particularly true in the case of long-term solvent exposure, solvent abuse and drug abuse. Despite these caveats, however, neuroimaging techniques provide a unique research tool with which to investigate structural and biochemical changes in neurotoxic disease and, in the future, may constitute an important source of information regarding structural and functional changes in the human brain as a function of neurotoxic exposures.

4.3 Types of human studies

Well documented human neurotoxicology studies have an advantage over studies in animals, in that human studies provide the most relevant information on neurotoxic effects in the species of concern. Human studies also provide a framework for identifying hazards in humans in the context of concomitant risk factors and individual differences in susceptibility (IPCS, 1999).

There are a number of different types of human studies that have been used to investigate the effects of neurotoxicants in humans, including case reports, population-based epidemiological studies and experimental exposure studies.

4.3.1 Clinical case-studies

Quite often the first information available to raise a level of concern for a health-related incident is a single case report or a cluster of cases indicating increased incidence of an adverse health effect. These reports may identify instances of a disease and are reported by clinicians or discerned through active or passive surveillance, usually in the workplace.

In the workplace, the occurrence of a particular neurotoxic disease in an appropriate occupational setting may constitute what is called a sentinel health event (SHE). Some examples of neurotoxic SHEs include toxic encephalopathy due to lead exposure in foundry workers, ship repair workers and bridge demolition workers; Parkinson's disease due to manganese exposure in workers involved in manganese mining, steel manufacturing and welding or to carbon disulfide exposure in workers in the rayon industry; cerebellar ataxia due to organic mercury exposure in fungicide manufacturing; and peripheral neuropathy due to exposure to *n*-hexane, methyl *n*-butyl ketone or other solvents in workers in the furniture refinishing industry, plastic-coated fabrics manufacture and paint manufacture (Ford et al., 1994). Because of the specificity of effects with these particular exposures, the occurrence of even a single case should alert physicians to the possibility of a neurotoxic disease.

In most instances, individual case-studies report the symptoms of individual patients who do not have a clear-cut history of type and level of neurotoxic exposure. Thus, despite the important role that clinical reports have played in helping to document the occurrence of different neurotoxic diseases, they are of only limited value in hazard identification in the risk assessment process. This is due to their often anecdotal nature, the small number of cases involved in most reports, the lack of statistical analysis and the difficulties in determining the exact type and level of exposure. Further, clinical evaluations may be performed quite differently by different physicians, and it is often difficult to judge exactly how the physical examination was performed or the reliability of the different procedures (Longstreth et al., 1994).

In spite of these limitations, clinical studies of individual patients can play a seminal role in helping to formulate hypotheses for testing in more controlled studies. Careful case histories can help to identify common risk factors, especially when the association between the exposure and disease is strong, the mode of action of the agent is biologically plausible, and clusters occur in a limited period of time. Moreover, the effects seen in patients at high levels of exposure may suggest possible approaches for examining the effects of long-term, low-level exposure in field studies of exposed populations or in acute experimental exposure studies.

4.3.2 Epidemiological studies

The purpose of epidemiological studies in neurotoxicology is the investigation of causal relationships between exposure and the occurrence of neurological disease. Many different study designs are available to examine the relationship between exposure and the occurrence of disease in epidemiological studies. Each study design type has strengths and weaknesses, which have been described in detail elsewhere (see Rothman & Greenland, 1998). Recent reviews of the different types of epidemiological studies in neurotoxicology are also available (Valciukas, 1991; Longstreth et al., 1994; Checkoway & Cullen, 1998). Guidelines for conducting environmental epidemiology studies have also been published (WHO, 2000).

In epidemiological studies, measures of disease frequency are reported in terms of prevalence and incidence. Prevalence refers to the proportion of individuals who are affected at a given time, while incidence is a measure of the new cases of a particular disease. In order to use incidence as a measure of disease frequency, it is necessary to take into account the time elapsed before disease occurs as well as the period of time during which the events are counted. Typically, an incidence rate is calculated by using a denominator that represents the sum of time that each person was at risk for developing the disease, or person-time at risk, in order to obtain a measure of cumulative frequency (Longstreth et al., 1994; Rothman & Greenland, 1998). In general, the incidence and prevalence are related by the average duration of the disease, such that the product of the incidence and the average duration of disease is approximately equal to the prevalence.

For the purpose of discussion, epidemiological studies may be classified as either descriptive or analytic. The presence of a hypothesis typically differentiates the two. In descriptive studies, the frequency of disease and the character of the population are documented. Case reports, for example, are descriptive in nature and are the simplest type of clinical epidemiological study (Longstreth et al., 1994).

Analytic epidemiological studies may be either observational or experimental. In experimental studies, the investigator has some control over the exposure and can allocate study participants using some form of randomization. Although experimental epidemiological studies are common in clinical epidemiology — namely, in randomized control clinical trials — such studies are, for obvious reasons, rare in neurotoxicology.

Observational study designs are, by far, the most common means of collecting data on the causal relationship between exposure and health effects in human neurotoxicity studies. Many types of observational study designs exist (Longstreth et al., 1994; Checkoway & Cullen, 1998; Rothman & Greenland, 1998). A discussion of several of these study designs is presented below.

The most frequently used observational design in neurotoxicology is the cross-sectional study. This approach involves sampling subjects on the basis of their level of exposure and comparing health end-points among groups. Cross-sectional studies are increasingly being used to monitor the health of workers to detect early neurotoxic effects, which are likely to be reversible in nature. The methods used often include a battery of neuropsychological tests, symptom questionnaires, behavioural physiological measures and electrophysiological assessments.

Cross-sectional studies limit the examination of exposed persons to a single point in time. However, a more comprehensive evaluation of the association between exposure and disease can be obtained using a longitudinal study design, in which effects testing and exposure assessments are repeatedly performed. In a longitudinal study, changes in reported symptoms and objective measures of neurological function can be examined over time in relation to exposure. By combining the cross-sectional and longitudinal study designs, changes in functional measures as a result of repeated testing can be adequately controlled for. Although longitudinal designs share the same limitations as cross-sectional designs (see below), they have the advantage that they provide information as to the permanence or reversibility of effects as a function of changes in exposure. Moreover, if subtle effects are found between exposed and non-exposed workers on only a few measures, repeated testing allows for an examination of the reliability of the effect on a particular measure.

There are a number of difficulties in the conduct and interpretation of cross-sectional studies. The aim of most occupational studies is to detect early, reversible effects to reduce or eliminate exposures. Typically, a large number of end-points from different functional domains are sampled in order not to overlook any changes that might be occurring. Because of the large number of end-points sampled, however, several significant effects can be expected to occur by chance alone. The decision to reject or accept the statistically significant effects for only several end-points as evidence of neurotoxicity in such cases is a matter of judgement and depends, to a large degree, on what is known regarding the compound, the power of the tests being used and the relationship of the severity of effects to exposure levels. Further, many of the functional tests used to assess neurotoxicity, including neurobehavioural tests as well as electrophysiological measures, may be affected by a host of factors unrelated to exposure (see Table 5). Thus, efforts must be taken to control for differences, preferably by matching subjects in the exposed and non-exposed groups on relevant variables that might affect study outcome. A final difficulty in occupational cross-sectional studies is the operation of the "healthy worker survivor effect" (Arrighi & Hertz-Picciotto, 1994). The healthy worker survivor effect refers to the continual selection process, whereby persons who remain employed tend to be healthier than those who leave employment. The healthy worker survivor effect tends to attenuate an adverse effect of exposure and, in practical terms, tends to be more problematic when evaluating subtle effects. Cross-sectional studies are often conducted for the purpose of surveillance of exposed workers with the aim of preventing neurotoxic disease in an exposed population. With prevention as the primary goal, cross-sectional studies can play an important role despite these limitations. In terms of risk assessment of individual compounds, however, cross-sectional studies are considered to provide relatively weak evidence with respect to the causal relationship between exposure and effect. To address issues of causality, two very powerful epidemiological designs are available: case–control studies and cohort studies.

A case–control study is an observational study in which persons are identified on the basis of the presence (cases) or absence (control) of a disease or other outcome variable of interest (Last, 1986). The cases and controls are selected from the same, clearly defined population, sometimes referred to as the source population. Information is then obtained regarding past exposures suspected of being risk factors for the disease or neurological dysfunction. In this sense, the collection of data is retrospective. The case–control study design allows an assessment of the association between disease or health effect occurrence and the level of exposure suspected of causing this effect. The relative frequency of the exposure (or potential risk factor) in both study groups serves as an estimate of the strength of association between the disease or outcome variable of interest and exposure level. Problems can arise in case–control studies because of bias in the selection of cases and controls and the possible differential recall of exposures between the two study groups.

The conduct of cohort studies can be either retrospective or prospective. The prospective cohort study is the closest to an experimental design, except that subjects, of course, are not randomly assigned to be exposed or not. In a prospective study, two or more groups of people or cohorts are identified who are free of disease, but differ with respect to their exposure to a toxic agent suspected of causing a particular disease (Rothman & Greenland, 1998). These cohorts are then followed over time for the development of the disease or diseases of interest. In the retrospective cohort study, the investigator has access to information on the cohorts collected at some time in the past and reconstructs the information on the cohorts regarding exposures and disease outcomes. A major difficulty with cohort studies relates to how quickly and how frequently the disease(s) of interest develop. If a disease is rare, prospective cohort studies are extremely difficult to do, because they require very large numbers of individuals who must be followed for long periods of time, especially when there is a latent period between exposure and disease onset. For this reason, they are less commonly used than case–control studies.

In order to use the data collected in case–control and cohort studies, a quantitative index must be computed to express the occurrence of the disease or outcome variable in relation to exposure. In cohort studies, the cumulative incidence of the disease in the exposed and control cohorts can be calculated for this purpose. The ratio of these incidences for exposed and control groups can then be used as a measure of the effect of exposure or relative risk. In the instance of a case–control study, this is typically computed by deriving an odds ratio, which is defined as the odds of exposure in the cases divided by the odds of exposure in the controls. When the disease or outcome variable is rare, the odds ratio is a reasonable estimate of relative risk.

A relative risk of 1 indicates that the exposure does not increase the risk of disease. As the relative risk increases beyond 1, the risk of disease associated with exposure increases. Thus, a relative risk of 2 would indicate that an exposed person would be twice as likely to develop a given disease as a non-exposed person. Relative risks can also fall between 0 and 1, in which case exposure is associated with a reduced risk of disease. Calculation of confidence intervals for measures of relative risk can provide estimates of their precision.

3.2.1   Assessment of exposure and dose

1)   Exposure assessment techniques

There are a number of different approaches to assess exposure in epidemiological studies (Armstrong et al., 1992). Examples of some of these are listed in Table 6. Also indicated is whether the technique is subjective or objective in nature and whether it can provide information regarding currently occurring or past exposures.

Table 6. Examples of methods of exposure and dose measurement in epidemiological studies[a]

Measurement methods	Data type		Time frame	
	Subjective	Objective	Present	Past
Personal interview	+	–	+	+
Checklist/simple questionnaires	+	–	+	+
Job exposure matrix (JEM)	+	–	+	+
Job-specific questionnaires	+	–	+	+
Diary	+	–	+	–
Observation by investigator	–	+	+	–
Measurements in the external environment	–	+	+	–
Reference to records	–	+	+	+
Measurements of internal concentrations	–	+	+	–
Biochemical markers	–	+	+	–

[a] Adapted from Armstrong et al. (1992).

As the table shows, many of the methods for assessing exposure are subjective in nature. Exposure information is obtained either by interview or by questionnaire. The personal interview is the most commonly used method in general epidemiology for obtaining data regarding environmental exposures. It allows information to be obtained on both present and past exposures, although both are subject to errors of recall. Exposed subjects tend to recall episodes of exposure extending outside of the time period of interest, leading to over-reporting. Likewise, underreporting of exposure may also occur in control subjects. The conduct of personal interviews is a costly and time-consuming method. Further, because it involves interaction between the study participant and the investigator, this method is also subject to the introduction of bias by the interviewer. Despite these disadvantages, the interview allows for more detailed and complex data than those afforded by other methods.

Data that can be collected by interview can, at least theoretically, be obtained by self-administered questionnaire. The use of questionnaires is probably the most simple and cost-effective means of assessing exposure and is typical in occupational epidemiology. Traditionally, investigators have used simple self-administered questionnaires or checklists to collect information regarding job title, type of industry and amount of time at different jobs. These data are then used to classify individuals on the basis of their degree of exposure. A related approach to exposure assessment is the job exposure matrix (JEM) method. This method involves the development of a database regarding the degree and type of exposure associated with different job titles in different industries. From the information obtained from the study subject on job title, duration, etc., the JEM is then used to help estimate the degree of specific exposures (e.g., Plato & Steineck, 1993). One of the limitations of the JEM method is that exposures may vary widely from worker to worker within the same job title, thus producing errors in individual estimates of exposure. To help improve the accuracy of exposure assessment, detailed job-specific questionnaires have also been developed.

Although the methods described above have been used in occupational toxicology for some time, there are surprisingly few studies that have assessed how well people can accurately report historical exposure information or whether the information can be accurately translated into accurate measurements of exposure (Stewart, 1999). Results from a recent study comparing these different subjective methods with an objective "gold standard" of environmental and biological monitoring data (Tielemans et al., 1999) indicate that measures of agreement among the different methods (i.e., simple checklists, JEM and the job-specific questionnaire) are generally poor to moderate. Results of this study indicated that data obtained with the job-specific questionnaire agreed better with analytical measures of internal exposure (i.e., biological monitoring data) than did data obtained with more traditional methods. One of the disadvantages of the job-specific questionnaire is that, compared with the other methods, the technique is time-consuming and costly. One approach proposed by Stewart (1999) is to use JEMs in studies of an exploratory nature and the more reliable job-specific questionnaire approach in studies designed to examine a causal relationship between exposure and health effects.

In addition to subjective methods used in exposure assessment studies, several objective approaches are also available for measuring exposure. Two of the most commonly used approaches are environmental monitoring (e.g., the measurement of chemicals in the environment) and biomonitoring (i.e., the measurement of chemicals or their metabolites in exposed individuals). In addition, several biochemical markers of early effects are also available for assessing direct exposure (IPCS, 1999).

Industrial hygiene evaluation typically includes the measurement of chemicals in the workplace environment, which can be used as a measure of exposure. The industrial hygiene standard for measuring a worker's external inhalation exposure to a chemical is the personal air sampling approach (Ford et al., 1994). The most common classes of sampling devices are pump-based sampling trains and direct-reading devices. Pump-based sampling integrates the fluctuating chemical concentrations present in the external environment over a particular period of time, usually 8 h. The resulting measurement is referred to as the 8-h time-weighted average. Direct-reading instruments are called grab samples. These instruments are typically used to measure peak concentrations in the external environment. Measurements of exposure in the workplace environment conducted at the time of the study provide information regarding present levels of ongoing ambient exposure, not past exposure. However, in occupational toxicology, records of measures made previously are sometimes available for inclusion in the overall estimate of exposure severity.

Occupational exposure limits are based on the airborne concentrations of chemicals in the workplace. However, exposure through the skin or through ingestion is also possible. Depending on the work environment, the work duties of individual workers and personal hygiene factors, the absorbed dose of a chemical can vary significantly from person to person in a given environment. Further, individual differences in the metabolism of compounds may also lead to different internal levels of exposure. As a result, the measurement of internal levels of the parent compound or its metabolites in exposed individuals provides a more direct assessment of exposure and dose than measurements of external levels of exposure. The choice of whether to measure the parent compound or one or more of its metabolites depends upon the toxicological mechanism of action. One example in neurotoxicology is the use of biological monitoring of *n*-hexane. *n*-Hexane is metabolized to 2,5-hexanedione, which is the proximal cause of hexane-induced polyneuropathy. Thus, the measurement of 2,5-hexanedione is more informative than the measurement of *n*-hexane for monitoring exposure levels.

Occupational exposure limits based on biological monitoring of internal levels have been published for a wide variety of chemicals and recently reviewed for neurotoxicants (Maroni & Catenacci, 1994). Similar to environmental monitoring, biological monitoring data reflect present-day, ongoing exposure, and rarely are sufficient historical records of biological monitoring data available to construct an integrated measure of exposure over time. As a result, the available data collected with these methods are typically integrated with data collected by questionnaire in order to provide estimates of exposure severity.

As internal levels of exposure to a neurotoxicant cannot be measured in the target tissue in humans, measurements in other biological tissues, such as blood or urine, are typically used to provide an estimate of exposure. In addition, several other media have also been employed. For example, measurements of metal concentrations in dentine pulp or hair can provide an estimate of exposure that reflects prior or cumulative exposure rather than recent exposure. In addition, hair can be sectioned to provide a temporal pattern of exposure as well. The major disadvantage of using hair as a medium in the occupational setting is the difficulty in distinguishing external contamination from internal incorporation. Further, body burdens of heavy metals in bone and soft tissue can also be measured using *in vivo* X-ray fluorescence (Ford et al., 1994). Care must be taken in comparing values of internal levels of exposure based on different tissues. Concentrations of lead in blood, for example, reflect most recent exposure, while bone lead reflects exposures over long periods of time.

The interpretation of biomonitoring data can be significantly enhanced by the use of mathematical models to describe the kinetics of the formation and elimination of toxic compounds and their metabolites (IPCS, 1993). Multicompartmental models for many biomarkers of exposure are well established and can be used to predict body burdens of chemicals in individuals and in communities.

Physiologically based pharmacokinetic (PBPK) modelling techniques may also prove useful in helping to estimate the severity of exposure or reconstruct internal levels of exposure based on environmental monitoring data. Briefly, a PBPK model is a set of mathematical equations that can be used to calculate the time course of the disposition of a xenobiotic in different anatomical compartments, including the target organ. Each anatomical compartment (e.g., liver, muscle, brain) has a characteristic blood flow, volume, tissue–blood partition coefficient and metabolic or clearance rate constant that together are responsible for a chemical's disposition in that region (Krishnan & Andersen, 1994). With the use of a PBPK model, one can predict the concentration of chemicals in different organs, including human brain, for different exposure scenarios, including peak exposures. If one had, for example, present-day and historical environmental sampling data for a particular compound and a validated PBPK model, it would be possible to estimate concentrations of the compound in human brain for those two exposure scenarios. Using this approach, it may be possible to obtain better estimates of internal body burdens of toxic chemicals occurring in the past, even if the half-life of the compound is quite short.

In addition to measures of body burdens of chemicals, early, presumably non-adverse, biochemical markers of effects can also serve as indices of exposure (IPCS, 1993; Ford et al., 1994; Costa & Manzo, 1998). These markers should identify early and reversible biochemical events, which may be predictive of later responses. Because biochemical measures of effects within the nervous system are impossible, surrogate markers for the CNS and PNS in readily accessible tissues are necessary.

One strategy has focused on the measurement of markers of neurotransmission in suitable peripheral cell systems. The best example of this strategy is the measurement of red blood cell AChE as an indicator of exposure to organophosphorus pesticides. Red blood cell AChE is an adequate surrogate because of its sensitivity, specificity and accessibility for measurement. In contrast, plasma cholinesterase can be influenced by a number of other factors, making it a less reliable marker.

Up until now, very few specific neurotoxicity biomarkers of effect have been developed; because of the inherent complexity of the nervous system, it is unlikely that general neurotoxicity markers will be developed (Costa & Manzo, 1998). In addition, the mechanism of action for most neurotoxic compounds is unknown, making progress in this field difficult. However, in cases where the molecular and cellular targets are known (e.g., organophosphates), useful biomarkers have been developed. Thus, for human biomarker research to progress, mechanistic studies elucidating the targets and mechanisms of action will be necessary.

2) Quantifying exposure and dose in human epidemiological studies

In order to obtain a quantitative estimate of the severity of exposure in epidemiological studies, a numerical index combining information regarding the level and duration of exposure is necessary. Cumulative exposure (average intensity × duration) is one of the most common summary measures for exposure, especially in occupational epidemiology (Ford et al., 1994). The index of cumulative exposure may be based on simple measures such as answers to questions regarding job titles as an estimate of average intensity multiplied by the number of years worked. On the other hand, estimates of cumulative exposure may also be quite complex, integrating, for example, present-day environmental levels of exposure measured using personal sampling techniques, company records of previous exposure levels associated with activities, and job-specific information during the person's working life.

Depending on the type of information obtained in the exposure assessment, exposure can be characterized as dichotomous (e.g., exposed versus non-exposed), ranked according to degree of severity (e.g., low, medium and high exposure) or expressed as a continuous variable. The dichotomous exposure characterization is the simplest exposure characterization. Although such a characterization may be useful in descriptive epidemiological studies, the heterogeneity of exposure characteristics for the different individuals in the study typically contributes to what is known as random exposure misclassification. Random misclassification error tends to reduce the probability of finding a relation between exposure and a health effect. Exposure characterizations that take into account intensity of exposure reported by the individual study participants using checklists, questionnaires, etc. coupled with exposure measurements in the workplace are the minimal standard in occupational studies at this time (Ford et al.,

1994). However, these methods, too, are subject to errors of exposure misclassification, which can seriously threaten the validity of epidemiological studies (e.g., Flegal et al., 1991).

Studies in the field of neurotoxicology have been criticized for the quality of exposure data reported (Stephens & Barker, 1998). It is of utmost importance to develop a strategy for characterizing the severity of exposure in the conduct of epidemiological neurotoxicity studies. Without evidence of dose–effect relationships, it is virtually impossible to infer a causal link between exposure and effect.

4.3.2.2 Causal inferences and confounding factors

To infer a causal relationship between a given exposure and neurotoxicity, the results of individual reports need to be critically evaluated. Individual studies should be examined for exposure data, the health outcome under study, the size of the study population, the control of possible confounders and the statistical power of the methods used to detect adverse effects. Studies that are negative — i.e., studies in which no effects of exposure are found — need to be carefully examined, particularly for study power and exposure misclassification. Power can be enhanced by combining populations from several studies using a meta-analysis (Bletner, 1999).

There is no clear-cut criterion to distinguish positive from negative studies. Although statistical significance is the gold standard in animal and human experimental studies, many epidemiologists consider such a view to be overly simplistic (Rothman & Greenland, 1998; IPCS, 1999). For example, the finding of a not statistically significant relationship between exposure and the outcome variable in epidemiological studies may simply reflect inadequate sample size or some other aspect of the study design. Conversely, when the results of a study are statistically significant, the seemingly positive results may still be due to unrecognized confounding or other bias.

Bias may result from study group selection or methods of data collection (Rothman, 1988). Information bias can result from misclassification of characteristics of individuals or events identified for study. This may include recall bias or interview bias. Studies with a low probability of biased data should carry more weight.

In fact, rarely does a single human study provide adequate evidence to establish a causal relationship between exposure and health effects. It is when several different studies, employing different study designs, demonstrate consistent results that the hypothesis of causality is best supported. A set of criteria for assessing the weight of evidence for causality based on the assessment of the epidemiological database has been developed (Hill, 1965). These criteria, in the context of neurotoxicology studies, are discussed below:

1) *Strength of the association measured by relative risk:* Hill (1965) argued that strong associations are more likely to be causal than weak ones, and, in general, epidemiologists have more confidence in their results when their findings indicate that the relative risk is large. However, relative risks of small magnitude do not necessarily imply the lack of causality. This is particularly important if the neurotoxic disease under study is relatively common (e.g., polyneuropathy) or is multifactorial in nature (e.g., dementia) (Rothman & Greenland, 1998; IPCS, 1999).

2) *Consistency of the association:* As mentioned above, the reproducibility of findings by different investigators using different populations and study designs constitutes one of the strongest arguments for the existence of causality. If there are discordant results, possible reasons should be considered in assessing the results, and data from studies considered to be of high quality should be given greater weight than data from methodologically less sound studies. A formalized method for this process is meta-analysis, by which pertinent epidemiological or clinical studies fulfilling basic requirements in terms of internal validity are combined to arrive at collective estimates of the strength of the association between exposure and effect not available from the individual studies within the set. An example in this respect is the meta-analysis of cross-sectional and cohort studies on the association between environmental lead exposure and psychometric intelligence in children (Pocock et al., 1994).

3) *Temporal relationship between cause and effect:* This criterion requires that exposure to a neurotoxic agent must precede the neurotoxic effect. This criterion of a temporal relationship was recently used in the design of an epidemiological study aimed at elucidating the role of different exposures in unexplained illness

in US Gulf War veterans (Spencer et al., 1998). Results from this study revealed that illness among veterans was not a function of the period of time they were actually present in the theatre of operations. That is, illness was distributed to the same degree in persons who served prior to, during and following the actual conflict, thus arguing against exposure to a neurotoxic agent as the cause of the illness.

4) *Biological gradient of the association:* Evidence for causality is strengthened when the risk for disease is shown to increase with increased levels of exposure. However, because there are many reasons that an epidemiological study may fail to detect a linear exposure–effect or exposure–response relationship, the absence of a dose–response or dose–effect relationship does not necessarily imply that the relationship is not causal.

5) *Specificity of the association:* The specificity criterion requires that the disease under study is caused only by a particular agent or that a particular agent produces only a specific disease. Specificity of cause is common in infectious diseases, but much less so in chronic diseases with multifactorial causes (IPCS, 1999). In neurotoxicology, many examples of known neurotoxic disease exist (e.g., polyneuropathy due to *n*-hexane, acrylamide, etc.; parkinsonism due to manganese, MPTP, etc.) that are not specific to only one compound. Moreover, one of the features of neurotoxicity is the fact that not only does an effect on a particular endpoint become more severe as exposure increases, higher dose rates of exposure also tend to broaden the spectrum of effects seen (Weiss, 1988). For example, at low dose rates, paraesthesia may be the only sign of adult methylmercury toxicity. At higher dose rates, the latency to paraesthesia may be shortened and accompanied by permanent visual loss. With higher dose rates, the onset of effects may be again shortened and accompanied by ataxia. This feature of neurotoxicity may significantly complicate the interpretation of human studies, particularly if effects are subtle and no clear-cut dose–effect/response relationships can be established.

6) *Biological plausibility of the association:* An epidemiological inference of causality is strengthened by data from experimental studies showing consistency with biological mechanisms.

However, the lack of mechanistic or positive animal bioassay data to support an association observed in an epidemiological study is not, in itself, reason to reject the inference of causality (IPCS, 1999). Several examples in the neurotoxicology literature include the lack of a model in the rat for MPTP-induced parkinsonism, the lack of an animal behavioural model for solvent-induced toxic encephalopathy and the relative insensitivity of the rat to organo-phosphate-induced peripheral neuropathy.

4.3.3 Human experimental exposure studies

In addition to epidemiological studies, well conducted experimental exposure studies in humans are also an important source of information for neurotoxicity risk assessment. Human laboratory experiments involve short-duration exposures (i.e., 2–6 h) for one or several consecutive days by the inhalatory route using either a mask or a controlled environmental chamber. Because many organic solvents are regulated on the basis of acute effects (Kulig, 1996), most studies have been conducted to evaluate the effects of these compounds, often in conjunction with toxicokinetic studies (Dick, 1995). In a typical laboratory study, solvent concentrations in blood are measured before, during and following exposure, and effects on the nervous system are assessed using symptom ratings, behavioural performance tests or electrophysiological methods. Most studies have been conducted in subjects under non-workload (i.e., sedentary) conditions. However, several studies have attempted to introduce "peak exposures" by either incorporating a workload condition (i.e., physical exercise), which has the result of increasing internal blood levels of exposure, or introducing periods of fluctuating high exposure peaks. Table 7 lists some of the solvents that have been studied in human laboratory studies alone or in combination with other chemicals and drugs.

From a methodological standpoint, human laboratory studies can be divided into two categories: between-subject and within-subject designs. In the former, the performance of exposed volunteers is compared with that of non-exposed participants. In the latter, performance is measured in the same individuals under exposure and non-exposure conditions. Within-subject designs have the advantages of requiring fewer participants and of eliminating individual differences as a source of variability. A disadvantage of the within-subject design is that certain tests, including neurobehavioural tests, must be administered

Table 7. Solvents and combinations studied in human laboratory experiments[a]

■ acetone	■ perchloroethylene (PER) (tetra-
■ acetone and methyl ethyl	chloroethylene)
ketone (MEK)	■ PER and ethanol
■ carbon tetrachloride	■ PER and diazepam
■ Fluorocarbon 113	■ styrene
■ MEK	■ toluene
■ methyl chloride (chloro-	■ toluene and ethanol
methane)	■ toluene and MEK
■ methyl chloride and ethanol	■ toluene and xylene
■ methyl chloride and diazepam	■ trichloroethylene
■ methyl chloroform (1,1,1-tri-	■ trichloroethylene and ethanol
chloroethane)	■ trichloroethylene and
■ methylene chloride (dichloro-	meprobamate
methane)	■ trichloroethylene and
■ methyl isobutyl ketone (MIBK)	thonzylamine
■ MIBK and MEK	■ vinyl chloride
■ MIBK and toluene	■ white spirit
■ propylene glycol dinitrate (jet	■ xylene
fuel)	■ xylene and ethanol
	■ xylene and methyl chloroform

[a] From Dick (1995).

more than once. Since practice on some neurobehavioural tests often leads to improved performance, which may confound the effect of the chemical/drug, there should be a sufficient number of test sessions in the pre-exposure phase of the study to allow performance on all tests to achieve a relatively stable baseline level.

Participants in laboratory exposure studies may be recruited from populations of persons already exposed to the chemical (e.g., solvent workers) or from chemically naive populations. Chemically naive volunteers are often younger, healthier and better educated than those exposed in the workplace and therefore may be less vulnerable to neurotoxicants.

Compared with workplace and environmental exposures, laboratory exposure conditions can be controlled more precisely, but exposure periods are much shorter, and ethical considerations limit the dose that can be given. In addition, double-blind studies have been shown to provide some control for the observer bias that may occur in single-blind studies. More credence should be given to those studies in which both observer bias and subject bias are carefully controlled (Benignus, 1993).

4.3.4 Developmental human neurotoxicity studies

While adult neurotoxicology evaluates the effects of chemical exposure on relatively stable nervous system structure and function, developmental neurotoxicology addresses the special vulnerabilities of the young. Neurobehavioural assessment of chemical neurotoxicity is complicated by having to measure functional impairment within a sequential progression of emergence, maturation and the later gradual decline of nervous system capabilities (Landrigan et al., 2000).

Exposure of pregnant women to alcohol, recreational drugs, therapeutic drugs, nicotine and environmental chemicals may result in the immediate or delayed appearance of neurobehavioural impairment in children (Kimmel, 1988; Nelson, 1991a; Tilson, 1998a; Jacobson & Jacobson, 1999). Postnatal exposure of children to chemical agents in the environment, such as lead, also may impair IQ and other indices of neurobehavioural function (Needleman et al., 1990). Neurotoxic effects may impair speech and language, attention, general intelligence, "state" regulation and responsiveness to external stimulation, learning and memory, sensory and motor skills, visuospatial processing, affect and temperament, and responsiveness to non-verbal social stimuli. Chemical neurotoxicity may be manifested as decreases in functional capabilities or delays in normative developmental progression.

Neurobehavioural functions emerge during developmental phases from the neonatal stage through to adolescence, and nervous system insult may be reflected not only in impairment of emergent functions, but also as delays in the appearance of new functions. Both the severity and type of deficit are affected by the dose and duration of exposure (Nelson, 1991b), and different sensitivities to chemical effects may be exhibited at different stages of nervous system development. Early episodes of exposure may produce damage to the nervous system that may not be developmentally expressed in behaviour for several months or years (Harry, 1994; Weiss, 2000).

The end-points frequently used to assess developmental neurotoxicity in exposed children have been reviewed by Winneke (1995). Jacobson & Jacobson (1999) have reviewed methodological issues associated with the design of prospective, longitudinal developmental studies. These authors have divided the types of tests used in human developmental neurotoxicology into two categories: apical and narrow-band tests. Examples of apical tests are IQ tests and the Bayley Scales. In apical testing, successful performance on a single measure or subtest may depend on the integrity of the nervous system and motivational factors (Jacobson & Jacobson, 1999). Narrow-band tests focus on more specific changes in neural development, such as attention or memory.

The selection of appropriate testing methods and conditions is very important when assessing children because of their short attention spans and dependence on parental and environmental supports. In addition, because of the increasing complexity of functional capabilities during early development, only a few tests appropriate for infants can be validly readministered to older children. Another complication specific to developmental studies is the necessity to adequately include covariates known to influence human cognitive development over and above early exposure to neurotoxic chemicals. Prominent among these covariates are parental intelligence and the "quality of the home environment," as assessed by the "Home Observation for Measurement of the Environment = HOME" (Caldwell & Bradley, 1984). The importance of these variables has been demonstrated in prospective studies on the association between environmental lead exposure and intelligence (Bellinger, 1995).

In addition, assessment methods must take into consideration the time (days, months or years) that may intervene between exposure/insult and the expression of neurotoxicity as functional impairment and should include repeated administration across a significant portion of the life span. Further, while gender differences in early development have been noted, differential responses of males and females to neurotoxicants have been less well explored and should receive attention. Research on non-exposed populations to develop age-appropriate normative scores for neurobehavioural functions will be important for the interpretation of assessment instruments. Finally, to improve the comparability of studies, assessment methods will have to be adapted to diverse ethnic, cultural and language groups in a fashion similar to that used for the development of testing batteries in adults (Anger et al., 2000). Given the complexity of evaluating developmental neurotoxic effects, the task of devising sensitive, reliable and valid assessment instruments or batteries for paediatric populations will be challenging.

4.4 Ethical considerations in human studies

Ethical considerations are of paramount importance in human studies. Ethical concerns pervade all phases of a human study, from its design to the publication of results, and there is a wide variation in the social and legal requirements for the conduct of human studies in different countries. Many research institutions and governmental agencies use independent panels to review research proposals with regard to the ethics of the research proposed. In some countries, the rights of the study participants are safeguarded by law, and "informed consent" is a legal requirement. In contrast, requirements may be less strict in other countries.

Guidance documents for the conduct of clinical trials of pharmaceutical agents have recently been published (e.g., WHO, 1995), and internationally recognized Good Clinical Practice (GCP) guidelines have been developed (e.g., the EC Principles of Good Clinical Practice). The study approaches contained in GCP guidelines for pharmaceuticals are also applicable to human experimental neurotoxicology studies. However, international Good Epidemiological Practice guidelines have not yet been published. In all cases where scientific research involves human participants, ethical codes developed internationally (e.g., the Declaration of Helsinki) should be taken into consideration (IPCS, 1983).

In all human research studies, subjects should be carefully informed as to the overall nature of the study and given a detailed account of its procedures. Prospective participants must not be pressured into participation and should be able to withdraw from the study at any time, without prejudice. Benefits of the study to the participants or to society should far outweigh the risks, and the techniques used should not produce harmful effects. Further, individual results must be held in strict confidence and should not be released, even to a family physician, without the authorization of the participant. Confidentiality is critical, since employment and insurance opportunities may be denied the participant if abnormalities or markers of susceptibility are found and reported (IPCS, 1983, 1999).

The issue of confidentiality is a complicated and difficult one in epidemiological studies. Although the use of medical information can be discussed with the study participant in many studies, the study design in some epidemiological studies may call for the examination of case notes of large groups of patients, whereby no direct contact with individual patients is made. Even if relatively non-controversial information is being extracted, those extracting the data may see more sensitive information. Concern regarding confidentiality may also extend beyond medical records. For example, in studies of occupational disease, factory payrolls have often been used. Such information may be kept for long periods of time, and the information can enable a cohort study to be done in a retrospective way. Although access to such information may be of great value to the epidemiologist, this information was obtained without the employees being informed that it might be used. However, if the use of such lists were restricted, information regarding the health risks of particular occupations would be difficult, if not impossible, to obtain.

4.5 Summary

There has been significant progress in the last decade in developing validated methods for detecting neurotoxicity in humans as well as an increased understanding of the factors that impact on the validity and reliability of human neurotoxicity studies. Standardized neuropsychological tests, validated computer-assisted test batteries, neurophysiological and biochemical tests, and refined imaging techniques have been improved for use in both clinical and research applications. These techniques are being utilized in different epidemiological study designs to examine the relationship between exposure to neurotoxic compounds and health effects.

Since the determination of exposure–response/effect relationships is a prerequisite for inferring a causal relationship between a chemical and a health effect, reliable and valid methods to determine the degree of exposure are of critical importance in these studies. Environmental monitoring can be used to measure current levels of external exposure, and biochemical techniques can be used to measure levels of internal exposure. Modelling techniques, such as PBPK modelling, may also prove useful in helping to interpret biomonitoring data. These objective measures, coupled with subject-specific information, can be used to provide estimates of dose. Recent studies, however, demonstrate the difficulties in obtaining reliable estimates of exposure and dose in human studies and highlight the need for improved methods in this area. In addition, the development of methods for measuring early biochemical effects (i.e., biomarkers of effect), which could be used to monitor early, readily reversible effects, should also be encouraged.

In addition, there are important individual differences in susceptibility to neurotoxic agents. The developing nervous system appears to be particularly vulnerable to some kinds of damage, and there is concern that neurotoxic exposure may be a contributory factor in neurodegenerative processes related to aging as well. Genetic differences in the metabolism of xenobiotics may also be of etiological importance in the expression of neurotoxic disease. Although progress has been made in the development of assessment techniques in children, more research is needed to establish normative data for use in different populations. Similarly, the study of the role of aging and genetic factors in the etiology of neurotoxic disease is also necessary.

5. ANIMAL NEUROTOXICITY

5.1 Animal models

5.1.1 Role of animal models

Determining the risk posed to human health from chemicals requires information about the potential toxicological hazards and the expected levels of exposure. Some toxicological data can be derived directly from humans. Sources of such information include accidental exposures to industrial chemicals, cases of food-related poisoning, epidemiological studies and clinical investigations. Although human data are available from clinical trials for therapeutics and provide the most direct means of determining effects of potentially toxic substances, it is usually not feasible to develop this type of information for other categories of substances. Quite often, the nature and extent of available human toxicological data are too incomplete to serve as the basis for an adequate assessment of potential health hazards. Furthermore, for a majority of chemical substances, human toxicological data are simply not available.

Consequently, for most toxicological assessments, it is necessary to rely on information derived from animal models, usually rats or mice. One of the primary functions of animal studies is to predict human toxicity prior to human exposure. In some cases, species phylogenetically more similar to humans, such as monkeys or baboons, are used in neurotoxicological studies.

Biologically, animals resemble humans in many ways and can often serve as adequate models for toxicity studies (Russell, 1991). This is particularly true with regard to the assessment of adverse effects on the nervous system, whereby animal models provide a variety of useful information that helps minimize exposure of humans to the risk of neurotoxicity. There are many approaches to testing for neurotoxicity, including whole-animal (*in vivo*) testing and tissue/cell culture (*in vitro*) testing.

At present, *in vivo* animal studies currently serve as the principal approach used to detect and characterize neurotoxic hazards and to help identify factors affecting susceptibility to neurotoxicity. Data from animal studies are used to supplement or clarify limited information obtained from clinical or epidemiological studies in humans and to provide specific types of information not readily obtainable from humans due to ethical considerations. Frequently, results from animal studies are used to guide the design of toxicological studies in humans.

In vitro studies have been proposed as a means of complementing whole-animal experiments. They appear to be most valuable when used to provide information on basic mechanistic processes in order to refine specific experimental questions to be addressed in the whole animal (Atterwill & Walum, 1989; Goldberg & Frazier, 1989; Harry et al., 1998). The currently available strategies for *in vitro* studies have certain limitations, including the inability to model neurobehavioural effects such as loss of memory or sensory dysfunction or to evaluate effectively the influence of organ system interactions (e.g., neuronal, endocrinological, immunological) on the development and expression of neurotoxicity.

In using animal models to predict neurotoxic risk in humans, it is important to understand that the biochemical and physiological mechanisms that underlie human neurological and psychological functions are often incompletely understood and, therefore, are difficult, if not impossible, to model exactly in animals. While this caveat does not preclude extrapolating the results of animal studies to humans, it does highlight the importance of using valid animal models in well designed experimental studies.

5.1.2 Special considerations in animal models

1.2.1 Dosing scenario

The dosing strategy used in experimental animal studies is an important variable in the development and expression of neurotoxicity. Some neurotoxicants can produce neurotoxicity following a single exposure, whereas others require repeated dosing (Xu et al., 1998). Repeated dosing represents the typical pattern of human exposure to many chemical substances, although much reported toxicity testing in animals involves acute or subacute exposures. Significant differences in response may occur when an acutely toxic quantity of material is administered over different exposure periods. For some neurotoxicants, the onset of neurotoxicity can occur immediately after dosing, whereas others may require time after exposure for the toxicity to develop. Repeated exposure may result in a progressive alteration in nervous system function or structure, while latent or residual effects may be discovered only in association with age-related changes or after suitable environmental or pharmacological challenge (MacPhail et al., 1983; Zenick, 1983). To ensure adequate assessment of neurotoxicity, study designs should include multiple dosing regimens, e.g., repeated exposure, with appropriate dose-to-response intervals of testing. Although it is often difficult to directly mimic the human exposure situation in animals, the dose, exposure route and duration used in animal models should be sufficiently similar to identify a potential hazard. With additional information and understanding of biological processes, extrapolation to humans should be possible. The conduct of neurotoxicological evaluations in studies utilizing excessively toxic doses can be considered (as in the case of potentially neuropathic organophosphates, where neuropathy may be seen only after severe intoxication). However, such studies should, in general, be avoided, particularly for neurobehavioural studies, as systemic toxicity may hamper interpretation of the data. It is important to remember that chemicals may display different profiles of effects at different points along the dose–response curve.

5.1.2.2   Species differences

A particularly important issue in neurotoxicology is that of species differences (Festing, 1991). For example, non-human primates are more sensitive than rats (Boyce et al., 1984) and mice (Heikkila et al., 1984) to the neurodegenerative effects of MPTP, a by-product in the illicit synthesis of a meperidine analogue (Langston et al., 1983). Rat strains also may be differentially sensitive to some neurotoxicants (Moser et al., 1991). Although it is preferred that more than one species be tested, the cost required for routine multispecies testing must be considered. Whenever possible, the choice of animal models should take into account differences in species with regard to pharmacokinetics, genetic composition and sensitivity to neurotoxic agents. Other factors such as gender of the test animal must be taken into consideration in neurotoxicological risk assessment. Some toxic substances may have a greater neurotoxicological effect in one gender (Squibb et al., 1981; Matthews et al., 1990). Thus, screening evaluations frequently require both male and female animals. Longitudinal studies that assess both genders at any stage of development address many of the problems associated with differentially sensitive populations.

1.2.3   Other factors

There are a number of other factors that should be considered in the design and interpretation of neurotoxicity studies using animal models (IPCS, 1986b; ECETOC, 1992; OECD, 1999). Design factors include such issues as using properly trained personnel to conduct the studies (as studies that require interaction between experimenter and animal demand special skills and experience), using appropriate numbers of animals per group to achieve reliable statistical significance and controlling the time-of-day variability. Time of testing relative to exposure is also important for assessing neurotoxic end-points such as behaviour, and experiments should be designed to generate a time course of effects, including recovery of function, if any. Housing is an important environmental design factor, because animals housed individually and animals housed in groups can respond differently to toxic agents. Temperature, as an experimental variable, may also affect the outcome of neurotoxicological studies. The responsiveness to some chemicals (e.g., triethyltin, methamphetamine) varies with ambient temperature and route of administration (Dyer & Howell, 1982). Some neurobiological end-points can be influenced by the body temperature of the animal (Dyer, 1987).

Because a variety of systemic physiological changes can influence neuronal functions, it is important to recognize that chemical-related neurotoxicity could result from treatment-induced physiological changes, such as altered nutritional state (IPCS, 1986b; ECETOC, 1992). What can appear to be specific neurotoxicological signs (e.g., abnormal gait) can result from non-specific causes such as peritoneal inflammation or kidney damage. Hence, such end-points need to be supported by others to confirm a neurotoxic action. As part of a neurotoxicological profile, correlative measures, such as relative and absolute organ weights, food and water consumption, and body weight and body weight gain, may be signs of physiological change associated with systemic toxicity and may be useful in determining the relative contribution of general toxicity.

5.1.2.4   Statistical considerations

Experimental designs for animal and human neurotoxicological studies are frequently complex, with two or more major variables (e.g., gender, time of testing) varying in any single experiment. In addition, such studies typically generate varying types of data, including continuous, dichotomous and rank order data. Where possible, sequential testing of the same animals during the experiment (within-subject design) may decrease variability in the study. Knowledge and experience in experimental design and statistical analyses are important. There are several key statistical concepts that should be understood in neurotoxicological studies (IPCS, 1986b; Gad, 1989). The power, or probability, of a study to detect a true effect is dependent on the size of the study group, the frequency of the outcome variable in the general population and the magnitude of effect to be identified. Statistical evaluation of a treatment-related effect involves the consideration of two factors or types of errors to be avoided. A Type I error refers to the attribution of an exposure-related neurotoxicological effect when none has occurred (false positive), whereas a Type II error refers to the failure to attribute an effect when an exposure-related effect has actually occurred (false negative).

Continuous data (i.e., magnitude, rate, amplitude), if found to be normally distributed, can be analysed with a general linear model using a grouping factor of dose and, if necessary, repeated measures across time. Post hoc comparisons between control and other treatment groups can be made following tests for overall significance. In the case of multiple end-points within a series of evaluations, correction for multiple observations might be necessary, depending on the test used.

Descriptive data (categorical) and rank data can be analysed using standard non-parametric techniques. In some cases, if it is believed that the data fit the linear model, the categorical data modelling procedure can be used for weighted least-squares estimation of parameters for a wide range of general linear models, including repeated-measures analyses. The weighted least-squares approach to categorical and rank data allows computation of statistics for testing the significance of sources of variation as reflected by the model. An excellent review of statistical principles and procedures has been written by Gad & Weil (1994).

1.2.5   Animal welfare issues

The use of animal models in neurotoxicology raises both general and specific concerns. Specific problems arise because some of the human conditions that need to be modelled in animals are inherently aversive or distressing. Two examples of these are sensory neuropathy produced by thallium and limbic system damage produced by tri-methyltin. It is important to remember that the adverse effects produced by neurotoxic chemicals can be just as distressing as the more obvious direct effects of surgical procedures. However, the three basic principles used to minimize animal suffering — i.e., reduction, refinement and replacement — can still be used to advantage in neuro-toxicity, as in other branches of toxicology.

The use of optimal experimental design and statistical analysis will help ensure that only appropriate numbers of animals are used to obtain necessary data. This will include design features such as the incorporation of simple behavioural end-points (e.g., functional obser-vations) into the structure of dose range-finding and lethality estima-tion studies wherever possible, rather than treating them as additional experiments. It is vital to ensure that animal care staff are well trained in the detection of signs of pain and distress in the species under study and that these signs do not go unrecorded or untreated. Refinement of end-points is also important; i.e., the use of more subtle, earlier and less stressful indices of neurotoxicity will often lead to more readily interpretable results, as well as to a reduction in animal suffering. The issue of replacement of animal tests by *in vitro* alternatives is dealt with in section 5.4. Although this is rarely possible in the initial investigative phase of hazard characterization, *in vitro* end-points may be devised once the underlying mechanism of the effect is understood.

5.2 End-points of neurotoxicity

5.2.1 Introduction

Neurotoxicity can be measured at multiple levels of organization, including neurochemical, anatomical, physiological or behavioural. The uncertainties associated with data from any end-point can often be greatly reduced if interpreted within the context of other neuro-toxicological measures and systemic toxicity end-points, particularly if such measures are taken concurrently. Studies that rely on only one type of end-point can often be very difficult to interpret. Neurotoxic effects that reflect an indirect effect secondary to systemic toxicities may also be considered adverse. Table 8 provides examples of potential end-points of neurotoxicity at the behavioural, physiological, chemical and structural levels. The interpretation of the indicators in Table 8 as being specifically neurotoxic is dependent on the dose at which such changes occur and the possibility that damage to other organ systems may contribute to or cause such changes indirectly.

5.2.2 Behavioural end-points

Neurotoxicants produce a wide array of functional deficits, including motor, sensory, and learning or memory dysfunction (Tilson & Mitchell, 1984; IPCS, 1986b; Kulig, 1996; Kulig et al., 1996). Many procedures have been devised to assess overt as well as rela-tively subtle changes in those functions — hence their applicability to the detection of neurotoxicity and hazard characterization. Many of the behavioural tests that have been developed and validated with well characterized neurotoxicants have been reviewed elsewhere (IPCS, 1986b; Cory-Slechta, 1989; Tilson, 1990a; Tilson et al., 1997). Exam-ples of such tests, the nervous system function being measured and neurotoxicants known to affect these measures are listed in Table 9.

Behaviour reflects the integration of the various functional com-ponents of the nervous system. Many methods can provide information for more than one category of function. Changes in behaviour can arise from a direct effect of a toxicant on the nervous system or indirectly from its effects on other physiological systems. Understand-ing the interrelationship between systemic toxicity and behavioural changes (e.g., the relationship between liver damage and motor

Table 8. Examples of potential end-points of neurotoxicity in animals

End-points	Examples
Behavioural	■ Absence or altered occurrence, magnitude or latency of sensorimotor reflex ■ Altered magnitude of neurological measurements, such as grip strength or hindlimb splay ■ Increases or decreases in motor activity ■ Changes in rate or temporal patterning of schedule-controlled behaviour ■ Changes in motor coordination, weakness, paralysis, abnormal movement or posture, tremor ■ Changes in ongoing performance ■ Changes in attention ■ Changes in touch, sight, sound, taste or smell sensations ■ Changes in learning and memory ■ Occurrence of seizures ■ Altered temporal development of behaviours or reflex responses ■ Abnormally repetitive behavioural patterns ■ Autonomic signs
Neurophysiological	■ Change in NCVs, amplitude, latency or refractory period of sensory or motor responses ■ Change in latency or amplitude of SEP ■ Change in EEG pattern or power spectrum ■ Change in brain blood flow
Neurochemical	■ Alterations in synthesis, release, uptake, degradation of neurotransmitters, proteins or enzymes ■ Alterations in second messenger associated signal transduction ■ Alterations in membrane-bound enzymes or receptors regulating neuronal activity ■ Decreases in brain AChE ■ Inhibition of neuropathy target enzyme (NTE) ■ Altered developmental patterns of neuro-chemical systems ■ Altered cell-specific markers (e.g., glial fibrillary acidic protein, or GFAP)
Structural	■ Gross changes in morphology, including brain weight ■ Discoloration of nerve tissue ■ Haemorrhage or oedema in nerve tissue ■ Accumulation, proliferation or rearrangement of specific structural elements ■ Loss of cells ■ Dilation or constriction of the ventricles

Table 9. Examples of tests to measure neurotoxicity and representative chemicals in animals

Representative function	Procedure	Agents
Neuromuscular		
Weakness	Grip strength, swimming endurance, suspension from rod, discriminative motor function, hindlimb splay	*n*-Hexane, methyl butyl ketone, carbaryl
Incoordination	Mid-air reflex, gait measurements	3-Acetylpyridine, ethanol
Tremor	Rating scale, spectral analysis	Type I pyrethroids, DDT, Lolitrem
Myoclonic spasms	Rating scale, spectral analysis	Strychnine, Type II pyrethroids
Sensory		
Auditory	Discriminated conditioning Reflex modification	Toluene Trimethyltin
Visual toxicity	Discriminated conditioning	Methylmercury
Somatosensory toxicity	Discriminated conditioning	Acrylamide
Pain sensitivity	Discriminated conditioning (titration), functional observational battery (FOB)	Parathion
Olfactory toxicity	Discriminated conditioning	Methyl bromide, 3-methylindole
Learning/memory		
Classical conditioning	Nictitating membrane Conditioned flavour aversion Passive avoidance Olfactory conditioning	Aluminium Carbaryl Trimethyltin, β,β'-iminodipropionitrile Neonatal trimethyltin
Operant conditioning	One-way avoidance Two-way avoidance Y-maze avoidance Biel water maze Morris water maze Radial arm maze Delayed matching to sample Repeated acquisition Visual discrimination	Chlordecone Neonatal lead Hypervitaminosis A Styrene DFP Trimethyltin DFP Carbaryl Lead

activity) is extremely important (ECETOC, 1992). The presence of systemic toxicity may complicate, but does not preclude, interpretation of behavioural changes as evidence of neurotoxicity. In addition, a number of behaviours (e.g., schedule-controlled behaviour) may require a motivational component (e.g., hunger) for successful completion of the task. In such cases, experimental paradigms specifically designed to assess the motivation of an animal during behaviour might be necessary to enable interpretation. Behavioural tests are generally quantitative and non-invasive. Thus, the same animal may be tested repeatedly during a toxicity study to provide detailed information about the presence or absence of effects, severity of effects, the onset and duration of effects, as well as recovery.

2.2.1 *Observational batteries*

Clinical observations are often included in toxicity protocols and include cage-side monitoring of animals, as well as handling of animals at the time of dosing or body weight determination (ECETOC, 1992). Clinical observations may indicate changes in motor function, arousal or emotional state or pharmacological effects, such as sedation or anaesthesia.

More structured, systematic examinations are often referred to as the functional observational battery (FOB) and are designed to detect and quantify major overt behavioural, physiological and neurological signs (Gad, 1982; Alder & Zbinden, 1983; Moser, 1989, 1997; O'Donoghue, 1989; Ladefoged et al., 1995; LeBel & Foss, 1996). FOBs are often used in conjunction with other measures of toxicity, neuropathology or neurophysiology (Mattsson & Albee, 1988). A number of batteries have been developed, each consisting of tests generally intended to evaluate various aspects of sensorimotor function (Tilson & Moser, 1992). Many FOB tests are essentially clinical neurological examinations that rate the presence or absence — and, in many cases, the severity — of specific neurological signs. Most FOBs have several components or tests. A typical FOB is summarized in Table 10 and evaluates several functional domains, including neuro-muscular (i.e., weakness, incoordination, gait and tremor), sensory (i.e., audition, vision and somatosensory) and autonomic (i.e., pupil response and salivation) function.

Table 10. Measures in a representative functional observational battery
(FOB) in rats

Home cage and open field	Manipulative	Physiological
Arousal	Approach response	Body temperature
Autonomic signs	Click response	Body weight
Convulsions, tremors	Foot splay	
Gait	Grip strength	
Mobility	Righting reflex	
Posture	Tail pinch response	
Rearing	Touch response	
Stereotypy		

The relevance of statistically significant test results from an FOB is judged according to the number of signs affected, the dose(s) at which effects are observed, the nature, severity and persistence of the effects, and their incidence relative to control animals (Ladefoged et al., 1995; US EPA, 1998a). In general, if only a few unrelated measures in the FOB are affected or the effects are unrelated to dose, the results may not be considered evidence of a neurotoxic effect. If several neurological signs are affected, but only at high dose and in conjunction with other overt signs of toxicity, including systemic toxicity, large decreases in body weight, decreases in body temperature or debilitation, there is less persuasive evidence of a direct neurotoxic effect. In cases where several related measures in a battery of tests are affected and the effects appear to be dose dependent, the data are considered to be evidence of a neurotoxic effect, especially in the absence of systemic toxicity. It has been suggested that FOB data should be grouped into one or more of several neurobiological domains, including neuromuscular (i.e., weakness, incoordination, abnormal movements, gait), sensory (i.e., auditory, visual, somatosensory) and autonomic (salivation, pupillary response) functions (Tilson & Moser, 1992). This statistical technique may be useful when separating changes that occur on the basis of chance or in conjunction with systemic toxicity from those treatment-related changes indicative of neurotoxic effects. This approach may also reduce the volume and heterogeneity of data and allow for separate statistical comparison for each domain to produce an effects profile (Ladefoged et al., 1995). In the case of the developing organism, chemicals may alter the maturation or appearance of sensorimotor reflexes. Significant alteration in or delay of such reflexes is evidence of a developmental neurotoxicant.

The major advantages of FOB tests are that they can be administered within the context of other ongoing toxicological tests and provide some indication of the possible neurological alterations produced by exposure. Potential problems include insufficient inter-observer reliability, difficulty in defining certain end-points and the tendency towards observer bias. The latter can be controlled by using observers unaware of the actual treatment of the subjects. Some FOB tests may not be very sensitive to agent-induced sensory loss (i.e., vision, audition) or alterations in cognitive or integrative processes such as learning and memory. FOB data may be used to trigger additional experiments.

Observable behavioural convulsions (epileptiform seizures) are sometimes seen in observational battery testing. Such effects could be indicative of an adverse effect on the nervous system, but should be interpreted with caution. Convulsive movements are variable in nature, but are characterized by rapid involuntary contractions of muscle groups, usually transient, often repeated and building up to a peak of severity. They may be restricted to just facial or individual limb muscles or rapidly progress to alternating contractions of all the major flexor and exterior muscle groups. In severe cases, a sustained muscle contraction with suspension of breathing may last 5–10 s.

Occasionally, other neurotoxic actions of compounds can mimic some convulsion-like behaviours, examples of this being the sometimes violent, but essentially voluntary, righting reactions shown by animals with impaired motor coordination. In other cases, convulsions or convulsion-like behaviours may be observed in animals that are otherwise severely compromised, moribund or near death. In such cases, convulsions might reflect an indirect effect of systemic toxicity and are less clearly indicative of primary neurotoxicity. As discussed in section 4.2.3, electrical recordings of brain activity could be used to determine specificity of effects on the nervous system. Sub-convulsive activity, which is recognizable as focal EEG spiking, may be associated with any motor signs and is often accompanied by immobility.

These events can reflect CNS activity comparable to that of epilepsy in humans and could be defined as neurotoxicity.

5.2.2.2 Motor activity

Motor activity represents a broad class of behaviours involving coordinated participation of sensory, motor and integrative processes (Ladefoged et al., 1995). Assessment of motor activity is non-invasive and has been used to evaluate the effects of acute and repeated exposure to neurotoxicants (MacPhail et al., 1989). An organism's level of activity can, however, be affected by many different types of toxic agents, including non-neurotoxic agents. Motor activity measurements have also been used in humans to evaluate disease states, including disorders of the nervous system (Goldstein & Stein, 1985). Motor activity has several advantages for testing — i.e., it can be tested non-invasively, its expression does not require motivational procedures and it can be measured by automated recording, which can provide objective and quantitative data (ECETOC, 1992; Ladefoged et al., 1995).

Motor activity is usually quantified as the frequency of movements over a period of time. The total counts generated during a test period will depend on the recording mechanism and size and configuration of the testing apparatus. In some cases, a transformation (e.g., square root) may be used to achieve a normal distribution of the data. In these cases, the transformed data, and not raw data, should be used for risk assessment purposes. The frequency of motor activity within a novel environment usually decreases with time (i.e., habituation) and is reported as the average number of counts occurring in each successive block of time.

Following developmental exposures, neurotoxic effects are often observed as a change in the ontogenetic profile or maturation of motor activity patterns. Frequently, developmental exposure to neurotoxic agents will produce an increase in motor activity that persists into adulthood or that results in changes in other behaviours. This type of effect is evidence of a neurotoxic effect. Like other organ systems, the nervous system may be differentially sensitive to toxicants in groups such as the young. For example, toxicants introduced to the developing nervous system may kill stem cells and thus cause profound effects on adult structure and function. Moreover, toxicants may have greater access to the developing nervous system before the BBB is completely formed or before metabolic detoxifying systems are functional.

Motor activity measurements are typically used with other tests (e.g., FOB) to help detect neurotoxic effects. Although changes in motor activity often occur at exposure levels that affect other classes of behaviour and at levels of exposure that do not produce gross signs of intoxication (Ladefoged et al., 1995), interpretation of motor activity data in isolation can be problematic. Agent-induced changes in motor activity associated with other overt signs of toxicity (e.g., loss of body weight, systemic toxicity) or occurring in non-dose-related fashion are of less concern than changes that are dose dependent, are related to structural or other functional changes in the nervous system or occur in the absence of life-threatening toxicity.

There are many different types of activity measurement devices, differing in size, shape and method of movement detection (MacPhail et al., 1989). Because of the accuracy and ease of calibration, devices with photocells are widely used. In general, situating the apparatus to minimize extraneous noise, movements or lights usually requires that the recording devices be placed in light- and sound-attenuating chambers during the testing period. A number of different factors, including age, gender and time of day, can affect motor activity and should be controlled or counterbalanced. Different strains of animals may have significantly different basal levels of activity, making comparisons across studies difficult. A major factor in activity studies is the duration of the testing session.

Motor activity can be altered by a number of experimental factors, including neurotoxic chemicals. Decreases in activity could occur following high doses of non-neurotoxic agents (Kotsonis & Klaassen, 1977; Landauer et al., 1984). If significant decreases in motor activity are seen, other contributing factors should be investigated. Examples of neurotoxic agents that decrease motor activity include many pesticides (e.g., carbamates, chlorinated hydrocarbons, organophosphates, pyrethroids), heavy metals (lead, tin, mercury) and other agents (3-acetylpyridine, acrylamide, 2,4-dithiobiuret). Some neurotoxicants (e.g., toluene, xylene, triadimefon) produce transient increases in activity by presumably stimulating neurotransmitter release, whereas others (e.g., trimethyltin) produce persistent increases in motor activity by destroying specific regions of the brain (e.g., hippocampus). Increases in motor activity are more likely than decreases to be a specific indicator of neurotoxicity.

5.2.2.3   Neuromotor function

Motor function tests are designed to detect specifically impaired motor performance, as distinct from changes in overall activity (Newland, 1995). Motor dysfunction is a common neurotoxic effect, and many different types of tests have been devised to measure time- and dose-dependent effects. Anger (1984) reported 14 motor effects of 89 substances, which were classified into four types: weakness, incoordination, tremor, and myoclonia or spasms. Specialized tests to assess weakness include measures of grip strength, swimming endurance, suspension from a hanging rod, discriminative motor function and hindlimb splay. Rotarod and gait assessments measure incoordination, whereas rating scales and spectral analysis techniques quantify tremor and other abnormal movements (Tilson & Mitchell, 1984; ECETOC, 1992; Ladefoged et al., 1995).

An example of a more complex procedure to assess motor function has been described by Newland (1988), who trained squirrel monkeys to hold a bar within specified limits (i.e., displacement) to receive positive reinforcement. The bar was also attached to a rotary device, which allowed measurement of manganese-induced tremor. Spectral analysis was used to characterize the tremor.

Incoordination and performance changes can be assessed with procedures that measure chemical-induced alterations in force (Fowler, 1987). The accuracy of performance may reflect neuromotor function and is sensitive to the debilitating effects of many psychoactive drugs (Walker et al., 1981; Newland, 1988). Gait, an index of coordination, has been measured in rats under standardized conditions and can be a sensitive indication of specific damage to the basal ganglia and motor cortex (Hruska et al., 1979), as well as damage to the spinal cord and PNS (Guyot et al., 1997).

Procedures to characterize chemical-induced motor dysfunction have been used extensively in neurotoxicology. Most require pre-exposure training (including alterations of motivational state) of experimental animals, but such tests might be useful, inasmuch as similar procedures are often used in assessing humans. Examples of neurotoxicants that affect neuromotor function are listed in Table 9.

2.2.4   *Sensory function*

Alterations in sensory processes (e.g., paraesthesia, visual, olfactory or auditory impairments) are frequently reported signs or symptoms in humans exposed to toxicants (Anger, 1984; Ladefoged et al., 1995; Dorman et al., 1997). Several approaches have been devised to measure sensory deficits (ECETOC, 1992; Maurissen, 1995; US EPA, 1998a). Data from tests of sensory function must be interpreted within the context of changes in body weight, body temperature and other physiological end-points. Furthermore, many tests assess the behavioural response of an animal to a specific sensory stimulus; such responses are usually motor movements that could be directly affected by chemical exposure. Thus, care must be taken to determine whether proper controls were included to eliminate the possibility that changes in response to a sensory stimulus may have been related to agent-induced motor dysfunction.

Several screening procedures have been devised to screen for overt sensory deficits. Many rely on orientation or the response of an animal to a stimulus. Such tests are usually included in the FOB used in screening (e.g., tail-pinch or click responses). Responses are usually recorded as being present, absent or changed in magnitude (Moser, 1989; O'Donoghue, 1989). Screening tests for sensory deficits are typically not suitable to characterize chemical-induced changes in acuity or fields of perception. The characterization of sensory deficits usually necessitates psychophysical methods that study the relationship between the physical dimensions of a stimulus and the behavioural response it generates (Maurissen, 1988).

One approach to the characterization of sensory function involves the use of reflex modification techniques (Crofton, 1990). Chemical-induced changes in the stimulus frequency or threshold required to inhibit a reflex are taken as possible changes in sensory function. Pre-pulse inhibition has also been used in neurotoxicology (Fechter & Young, 1983) and can be used to assess sensory function in humans as well as in experimental animals.

Various behavioural procedures require that a learned response occurs only in the presence of a specific stimulus (i.e., discriminated or conditioned responding). Chemical-induced changes in sensory function are determined by altering the physical characteristics of the stimulus (e.g., magnitude or frequency) and measuring the alteration in response rate or accuracy. In an example of the use of a discriminated conditional response to assess chemical-induced sensory dysfunction, Maurissen et al. (1983) trained monkeys to respond to the presence of a vibratory or electrical stimulus applied to the fingertip. Repeated dosing with acrylamide produced a persistent decrease in vibration sensitivity; sensitivity to electrical stimulation was unimpaired. That pattern of sensory dysfunction corresponded well to known sensory deficits in humans. Discriminated conditional response procedures have been used to assess the ototoxicity produced by toluene (Pryor et al., 1983) and the visual toxicity produced by methylmercury (Merigan, 1979).

Procedures to characterize chemical-induced sensory dysfunction have been used often in neurotoxicology. As in the case of most procedures designed to measure nervous system dysfunction, training and motivational factors can be confounding factors. Many tests designed to assess sensory function for laboratory animals can also be applied with some adaptation to humans. Examples of neurotoxicants that affect sensory function are listed in Table 9. Pain perception, as well as specific sensory modalities, can be altered by chemicals; for example, prenatal diazepam has been reported to modify stress-induced analgesia in rats (Muhammad & Kitchen, 1994). A variety of behavioural methods is available to study olfactory functions as endpoints of neurotoxicity. These range from simple homing responses in developmental studies to operant paradigms using psychophysical techniques in operant chambers (Wood, 1982). An overview of methods to assess olfactory function in a neurotoxicity context has been published by Hastings (1990).

5.2.2.5 Learning and memory

Laboratory animals possess cognitive functions that can be assessed by a number of techniques (Ladefoged et al., 1995). Alterations in learning or memory are often reported by adult humans as a consequence of toxic exposure (Anger, 1990a). Behavioural deficits in children have been caused by lead exposure (Smith et al., 1989), and it is hypothesized that chronic low-level exposure to toxic agents may have a role in the pathogenesis of senile dementia (Calne et al., 1986).

Learning can be defined as an enduring change in the mechanisms of behaviour that results from experience with environmental events (Domjan & Burkhard, 1986). Memory is a change that can be either short-lasting or long-lasting (Eckerman & Bushnell, 1992). Alterations in learning and memory must be inferred from changes in behaviour. However, changes in learning and memory must be separated from other changes in behaviour that do not involve cognitive or associative processes (e.g., motor function, sensory capabilities, motivational factors), and an apparent toxicant-induced change in learning or memory should be demonstrated over a range of stimuli and conditions (Tilson, 1997). It is well known that lesions in the brain can interfere with learning (Tilson, 1997). It is also known that some brain lesions can facilitate some types of learning by removing behavioural tendencies (e.g., inhibitory responses due to stress) that moderate the rate of learning under normal circumstances. A discussion of learning procedures and examples of chemicals that can affect learning and memory have appeared in reviews (Heise, 1984; IPCS, 1986b; Peele & Vincent, 1989; ECETOC, 1992; Tilson, 1997; US EPA, 1998a).

One approach to studying the effects of a chemical on learning and memory involves the pairing of a novel stimulus with a second stimulus that produces a known, observable and quantifiable response. The novel stimulus is known as the conditioned stimulus, and the second, eliciting stimulus is the unconditioned stimulus. With repeated pairings of the two stimuli, the conditioned stimulus comes to elicit a response similar to the response elicited by the unconditioned stimulus. The procedure has been used in behavioural pharmacology and, to a lesser extent, in neurotoxicology. Neurotoxicants that interfere with learning and memory would alter the number of presentations of the pair of stimuli required to produce conditioning or learning. Memory is tested by determining how long after the last presentation of the two stimuli the conditioned stimulus would still elicit a response (Yokel, 1983). Other classically conditioned responses known to be affected by psychoactive or neurotoxic agents are conditioned taste aversion (Riley & Tuck, 1985; Peele et al., 1990), conditioned suppression (Chiba & Ando, 1976), passive avoidance response (MacTutus et al., 1982; Shaughnessy et al., 1994) and the conditioned eye blink response (Stanton & Freeman, 1994).

Other procedures to assess learning or memory typically involve the pairing of a response with a stimulus that increases the probability of future response through reinforcement (Tilson, 1997). Response rate can be increased by using positive or negative reinforcement. Learning is usually assessed by determining the number of presentations or trials needed to produce a defined frequency of response. Memory can be defined specifically as the maintenance of a stated frequency of response after initial training. Neurotoxicants may adversely affect learning by increasing or decreasing the number of presentations required to achieve the designated criterion. Decrements in memory may be indicated by a decrease in the probability or frequency of a response at some time after initial training. Toxicant-induced changes in learning and memory should be interpreted within the context of possible toxicant-induced changes in sensory, motor and motivational factors (Tilson, 1997). Examples of instrumental learning procedures used in neurotoxicology are repeated acquisition (Schrot et al., 1984; Cohn et al., 1993) and two-way shuttle box avoidance (Tilson et al., 1987). Mazes, such as the Morris water maze, radial arm maze and Biel water maze, are being used with increasing frequency in neurotoxicology to assess spatial memory (Wirsching et al., 1984; Vorhees, 1985; Lee & Rabe, 1992; Barone et al., 1995). Other procedures using instrumental conditioning to assess neurotoxicity include delayed alternation, delayed matching to sample and discrimination reversal (Heise, 1984; Rice & Karpinski, 1988; Schantz et al., 1989; Bushnell et al., 1993). Examples of chemicals that affect learning and memory are listed in Table 9.

5.2.2.6 Attention

In order for learning to occur, the relationship between stimuli or between response and reinforcement has to be perceived or registered (Eckerman & Bushnell, 1992). Attention is fundamental to information processing, which occurs during the cognitive processes of learning and memory. It is not a unitary concept, but consists of several distinct mechanisms. Types or aspects of attention include sustained attention (vigilance), divided (distributed) attention and focused (selective) attention. Some typical experimental procedures for use in rats include Serial Reaction Performance, Post-Training Designs, Reaction Time Procedures, Discrimination Learning and Latent Inhibition models (Robbins et al., 1993). Examples of orienting include exploratory behaviour, response to novelty and signal detection, whereas stimulus anticipation and response preparation are examples of expectancy (Bushnell, 1998). The stimulus control in match-to-sample and spatial tracking are examples of stimulus differentiation, whereas sustained attention refers to the ability to report unpredictable stimuli over time. Parallel processing refers to the process required to perform a dual-task problem. The neurobiological substrate for attention is still being explored, but it appears that major neurotransmitters, such as the dopaminergic, adrenergic, cholinergic and GABA-ergic systems, are important for maintaining attention. Although effects of pharmacological agents on attention have been reported (Bushnell, 1998), little work has been done using neurotoxic chemicals (Eckerman & Bushnell, 1992).

2.2.7 *Schedule-controlled behaviour*

Schedule-controlled operant behaviour (SCOB) has been used extensively in psychopharmacology to quantify the effects of drugs on behaviour (Li, 1994). A schedule of reinforcement describes the relationship between a response and the consequences of the response, i.e., reinforcement or punishment. In many respects, maintenance of most behaviours made by humans and animals is under the control of various types of reinforcement contingencies and could be defined as schedule controlled. Sette (1994) points out that SCOB has been proposed as a routine screen for neurotoxicity, a paradigm that is triggered following results from hazard identification studies, to be used to characterize the effects of specific chemical classes, such as the acute effects of solvents, and in experiments involving repeated exposure for chemicals such as solvents that affect higher-order cognitive functions. Its use in neurotoxicology hazard identification has been limited.

In the laboratory, SCOB involves the maintenance of behaviour (e.g., performance of a lever press or key peck response) by the experimental manipulation of various contingencies of reinforcement known as schedules. Different rates and patterns of responding are controlled by the relationship between response and subsequent rein-forcement. SCOB provides a measure of performance of a learned behaviour (e.g., lever press or key peck) and involves training and motivational variables that must be considered in evaluating the data. Agents may interact with sensory processing, motor output, motiva-tional variables (i.e., related to reinforcement), training history and baseline characteristics (Rice, 1988; Cory-Slechta, 1989). Qualita-tively, rates and patterns of SCOB display cross-species generality, but the quantitative measures of rate and pattern of performance can vary within and between species.

In laboratory animals, SCOB has been used to study a wide range of neurotoxicants, including methylmercury, many pesticides, organic and inorganic lead, triethyltin and trimethyltin (MacPhail, 1985; Rice, 1988). The primary SCOB end-points for evaluation are response rate and the temporal pattern of responding. These end-points may vary as a function of the contingency between responding and reinforcement presentation (i.e., schedule of reinforcement). Schedules of reinforce-ment that have been used in toxicology studies include fixed ratio and fixed interval schedules. Fixed ratio schedules engender high rates of responding and a characteristic pause after delivery of each reinforce-ment. Fixed interval schedules engender a relatively low rate of responding during the initial portion of the interval and progressively higher rates near the end of the interval. For some schedules of reinforcement, the temporal pattern of responding may play a more important role in defining the performance characteristics than the rate of responding. For other schedules, the reverse may be true. For example, the temporal pattern of responding may be more important than rate of responding for defining performance on a fixed interval schedule. For a fixed ratio schedule, more importance might be placed on the rate of responding than on the post-reinforcement pause.

The overall qualitative patterns are important properties of the behaviour. Substantial qualitative changes in operant performance, such as elimination of characteristic response patterns, can be evidence of an adverse effect. Most chemicals, however, can disrupt operant behaviour at some dose, and such adverse effects may be due to either neurotoxic or non-neurotoxic mechanisms. Unlike large qualitative changes in operant performance, small quantitative changes in per-formance are not adverse. Some changes may actually represent an

improvement in performance, e.g., an increase in the index of cur-
vature with a decrease in fixed interval rate of responding. Assessing
the toxicological importance of these effects requires considerable
professional judgement and evaluation of converging evidence from
other types of toxicological end-points.

While most chemicals decrease the efficiency of responding at
some dose, some agents may increase response efficiency on schedules
requiring high response rates due to a stimulant effect or an increase
in CNS excitability. Agent-induced changes in responding between
reinforcements (i.e., the temporal pattern of responding) may occur
independently of changes in the overall rate of responding. Chemicals
may also affect the reaction time to respond following presentation of
a stimulus. Agent-induced changes in response rate or temporal
patterning associated with other overt signs of toxicity (e.g., body
weight loss, systemic toxicity or occurring in a non-dose-related
fashion) are of less concern than changes that are dose dependent, are
related to structural or other functional changes in the nervous system
or occur in the absence of life-threatening toxicity.

2.2.8   Pharmacological challenges

Pharmacological agents have been used frequently as challenges
in behavioural neurotoxicology, especially in animals that may have
been exposed to chemicals during development (Walsh & Tilson,
1986). This strategy is based on the premise that subtle alterations in
neurobiological processes may go unnoticed until the nervous system
is perturbed by factors such as drugs acting on it. It is known that the
nervous system can adapt to repeated perturbation, and exposure to
neurotoxic chemicals can alter the dynamic homeostatic processes
associated with normal functioning of the nervous system. However,
if the compromised nervous system is further challenged, as in the case
of exposure to psychoactive drugs, then the "functional reserve" of the
system will fail, and signs of nervous system deficits will be uncovered
or unmasked (Tilson & Mitchell, 1983). The use of pharmacological
challenges or probes in neurotoxicity assessments has at least two
advantages. First, it may help increase the sensitivity of behavioural
models to detect subtle nervous system alterations following exposure
to chemicals. Second, it may be useful to elucidate perturbations of

neurotransmitter systems that may underlie observed neurobehavioural changes due to chemical exposure (Walsh & Tilson, 1986).

D-Amphetamine is frequently employed as a pharmacological probe in neurotoxicological studies because its neurochemical and neural substrates are generally well known and its effects on various behaviours have been characterized. The use of D-amphetamine as a routine pharmacological challenge in studies involving developmental exposures has gained general acceptance. When there is evidence that the dopaminergic system is affected, a pharmacological challenge with D-amphetamine may unmask the effect either in the adult nervous system or following developmental exposure (Hughes & Sparber, 1978; Adams & Buelke-Sam, 1981; Buelke-Sam et al., 1985; Evangelista de Duffard et al., 1995a; Cory-Slechta et al., 1996).

Proconvulsant activity can be demonstrated by co-administration of the test agent with a subconvulsive dose of a convulsant such as picrotoxin. Shifts in the dose–response curve to the left or right in treated animals relative to controls support the conclusion of a compensatory change in nervous system sensitivity. However, other factors, such as differing pre-challenge baselines (Tilson et al., 1980) or pharmacokinetic factors (Robbins et al., 1978), must be ruled out before it can be concluded that a change in nervous system sensitivity has been unmasked by a pharmacological challenge. The choice of challenge is dependent upon the system suspected to be altered. Pharmacological challenges are best used when there are data available to determine the neurochemical system involved and pharmacological agent to employ. Physical challenges offer a slightly broader spectrum of uses, as a generalized stress response of the animal may "unmask" alterations in multiple target sites. Chemicals that have been shown to affect subsequent sensitivity to pharmacological challenge include carbon disulfide, acrylamide, lead, methylmercury, chlordecone and diisopropylfluorophosphate (Walsh & Tilson, 1986).

5.2.3 Neurophysiological end-points

Neurophysiological studies measure the electrical activity of the nervous system. The term "neurophysiology" is often used synonymously with "electrophysiology" (Dyer, 1987). Neurophysiological techniques provide information on the integrity of defined portions of the nervous system. Several neurophysiological procedures are available for application to neurotoxicological studies. Examples of neurophysiological end-points that could be used in neurotoxicity assessments are listed in Table 11 (Herr & Boyes, 1995). They range in scale from procedures that employ microelectrodes to study the function of single nerve cells or restricted portions of them to procedures that employ macroelectrodes to perform simultaneous recordings of the summed activity of many cells. Microelectrode procedures typically are used to study mechanisms of action and are frequently performed *in vitro*. Macroelectrode procedures are generally used in studies to detect or characterize the potential neurotoxic effects of agents of interest because of potential environmental exposure. The present discussion concentrates on macroelectrode neurophysiological procedures, because it is more likely that they will be the focus of decisions regarding critical effects in risk assessment. All of the procedures described below for use in animals have also been used in humans to determine chemically induced alterations in neurophysiological function.

Table 11. Potential neurophysiological measures of neurotoxicity

Name of end-point	Type of response
Electroretinograms	Evoked responses from the retina in response to visual stimuli
Flash visual evoked potentials (VEPs)	Cortical response to simple flashes of illumination
Pattern visual evoked potentials (VEPs)	Cortically generated responses elicited by patterns of visual stimuli
Brainstem auditory evoked potentials (BAEPs)	Responses recorded at or near the cortical surface reflecting volume-conducted electrical activity from brainstem generators in auditory pathway
Middle and late potentials	Potentials occurring in auditory cortex approximately 10–50 ms after auditory stimulation
"Far-field" somato-sensory evoked potentials (SSEPs)	Elicited by electrical stimulation of nerves, producing a large synchronous afferent volley in the CNS
Cortical somato-sensory potentials	Recorded from cerebral cortex after presentation of sensory stimuli or direct stimulation of the median nerve
Cerebellar somato-sensory potentials	Recorded from cerebellum after stimulation of peripheral nerve such as the ventral caudal tail nerve of rats

5.2.3.1   Peripheral nerve function studies

Nerve function studies, generally performed on peripheral nerves, can be useful in investigations of possible peripheral neuropathy. Most peripheral nerves contain mixtures of individual sensory and motor nerve fibres. It is possible to distinguish sensory from motor effects in peripheral nerve studies by measuring activity in sensory nerves or by measuring the muscle response evoked by nerve stimulation to measure motor effects (Ross & Lawhorn, 1990). EMG may also be used to study toxic neuropathies. While a number of end-points can be recorded, the most critical variables are (1) NCV, (2) amplitude of EPs and (3) refractory period. It is important to recognize that damage to nerve fibres may not be reflected in changes in these end-points if the damage is not sufficiently extensive. Thus, the interpretation of data from such studies may be enhanced if evaluations such as nerve pathology or other structural measures are also included.

Normal peak conduction measurements are influenced by a number of factors, the most important of which is temperature. An adequate nerve conduction study will either measure the temperature of the limb under study and mathematically adjust the results according to well established temperature factors or control limb temperature within narrow limits. Studies that measure peripheral nerve function without regard for temperature are not adequate for risk assessment.

A decrease in NCV may be indicative of demyelination. In cases where the primary toxic effect is axonal degeneration, NCV may not be reduced unless the fastest-conducting axons are affected (Ross et al., 1996). For this reason, a measurement of normal NCV does not necessarily rule out the presence of axonal degeneration.

Primary axonal degeneration may be reflected by decreases in peripheral nerve evoked response amplitude and may occur prior to or in the absence of conduction velocity in the course of peripheral neuropathy. Hence, changes in response amplitude may be more sensitive than conduction velocity as an index of axonal degeneration. However, measurements of response amplitude require careful application of experimental techniques (e.g., electrode positioning), a larger sample size and greater statistical power than measurements of velocity. The refractory period refers to the time required after stimulation before a nerve can fire again and provides a measure reflecting the functional status of nerve membrane ion channels.

In summary, alterations in peripheral NCV response amplitude and refractory period may help to detect or characterize neurotoxic effects. Alterations in peripheral nerve function are frequently associated with sensory or motor abnormalities such as tingling or weakness. Examples of compounds that alter peripheral nerve function in humans or experimental animals include acrylamide, carbon disulfide, *n*-hexane, lead and some organophosphates (Seppäläinen, 1998).

i.2.3.2   Sensory evoked potentials

EP studies are electrophysiological procedures that measure the response elicited from a defined stimulus such as a tone, a light or a brief electrical pulse. EPs reflect the function of the system under study, including visual, auditory or somatosensory; motor, involving motor nerves and innervated muscles; or other neural pathways in the CNS or PNS (Rebert, 1983; Mattsson & Albee, 1988; Boyes, 1992, 1993). EP studies should be interpreted with respect to the known or presumed neural generators of the responses and their likely relationships with behavioural outcomes, when such information is available. Such correlative information strengthens the confidence in electrophysiological outcomes. In the absence of such supportive information, the extent to which EP studies provide convincing evidence of neurotoxicity is a matter of professional judgement on a case-by-case basis. Judgements should consider the nature, magnitude and duration of such effects.

Data are in the form of a voltage record collected over time and can be quantified in several ways. Commonly, the latency (time from stimulus onset) and amplitude (voltage) of the positive and negative voltage peaks are identified and measured. Alternative measurement schemes may involve substitution of spectral phase or template shifts for peak latency and spectral power, spectral amplitude, root-mean-square or integrated area under the curve for peak amplitude. Latency measurements are dependent on both the velocity of nerve conduction and the time of synaptic transmission. Both of these factors depend on temperature, as discussed in regard to nerve conduction, and similar caveats apply for SEP studies. In studies that are well controlled for temperature, increases in latencies or related measures can reflect deficits in nerve conduction, including demyelination or delayed synaptic transmission, and are indicators of a neurotoxic effect.

Decreases in peak latencies, like increases in NCV, are unusual, but the neural systems under study in SEPs are complex, and situations that might cause a peak measurement to occur earlier are conceivable. Two such situations are a reduced threshold for spatial or temporal summation of afferent neural transmission and a selective loss of cells responding late in the peak, thus making the measured peak occur earlier. Decreases in peak latency should not be dismissed outright as experimental or statistical error, but should be examined carefully and perhaps replicated to assess possible neurotoxicity. A decrease in latency is not conclusive evidence of a neurotoxic effect.

Changes in peak amplitudes or equivalent measures reflect changes in the magnitude of the neural population responsive to stimulation. Both increases and decreases in amplitude are possible following exposure to chemicals. Whether excitatory or inhibitory neural activity is translated into a positive or negative deflection in the SEP is dependent on the physical orientation of the electrode with respect to the tissue generating the response, which is frequently unknown. Comparisons should be based on the absolute change in amplitude. Therefore, either increases or decreases in amplitude may be indicative of a neurotoxic effect.

Within any given sensory system, the neural circuits that generate various EP peaks differ as a function of peak latency. In general, early latency peaks reflect the transmission of afferent sensory information. Changes in either the latency or amplitude of these peaks are considered convincing evidence of a neurotoxic effect that is likely to be reflected in deficits in sensory perception. The later-latency peaks, in general, reflect not only the sensory input but also the more non-specific factors such as the behavioural state of the subject, including such factors as arousal level, habituation or sensitization (Dyer, 1987). Thus, changes in later-latency EP peaks must be interpreted in light of the behavioural status of the subject and would generally be considered evidence of a neurotoxic effect.

.2.3.3   Electroencephalography

EEG analysis is used widely in clinical settings for the diagnosis of neurological disorders and less often for the detection of subtle toxicant-induced dysfunction (IPCS, 1986b; Eccles, 1988; Ladefoged et al., 1995; Nagymajtenyi et al., 1995). The basis for using EEG in either setting is the relationship between specific patterns of EEG waveforms and specific behavioural states. Because states of alertness and stages of sleep are associated with distinct patterns of electrical activity in the brain, it is generally thought that arousal level can be evaluated by monitoring the EEG. Dissociation of EEG activity and behaviour can, however, occur after exposure to certain chemicals. Normal patterns of transition between sleep stages or between sleeping and waking states are known to remain disturbed for prolonged periods of time after exposure to some chemicals. Changes in the pattern of the EEG can be elicited by anaesthetic drugs and stimuli producing arousal (e.g., lights, sounds). In studies with toxicants, changes in EEG pattern can sometimes precede alterations in other objective signs of neurotoxicity (Dyer, 1987).

EEG studies must be done under highly controlled conditions, and the data must be considered on a study-by-study basis. Recordings of spontaneous EEG have not often been used in experimental animal toxicology.

.2.3.4   Seizure activity

Some neurotoxicants (e.g., lindane, pyrethroids, trimethyltin, dichlorodiphenyltrichloroethane) produce observable convulsions. When convulsion-like behaviours are observed, as described in section 5.2.2.1, neurophysiological recordings can provide additional information to help interpret the results. Recordings of brain electrical activity that demonstrate seizure-like activity are indicative of a neurotoxic effect.

In addition to producing seizures directly, chemicals may also alter the frequency, severity, duration or threshold for eliciting seizures (Joy et al., 1982). Such alterations can occur after acute exposure or after repeated exposure to dose levels below the acute seizure threshold. In experiments demonstrating changes in sensitivity following repeated exposures to the test compound, information regarding possible changes in the pharmacokinetic distribution of the compound is required before the seizure susceptibility changes can be interpreted as evidence of neurotoxicity. Increases in susceptibility to seizures are considered adverse.

5.2.3.5 Electromyography

EMG involves making electrical recordings from muscle and has been used extensively in human clinical studies in the diagnosis of certain diseases of the muscle and for detecting peripheral axonal impairments (He, 1985; IPCS, 1986b; He et al., 1989; Jabre, 1995). Changes in the EMG include amplitude and firing frequency of spontaneous firing; evoked muscle responses to nerve stimulation can be used to study alterations in a motor unit, which includes the alpha motor neuron, nerve root, peripheral nerve, neuromuscular junction and muscle. EMG has been used to study toxicant-induced changes in neuromuscular function, including organophosphate insecticides, methyl *n*-butyl ketone, and botulinum and tetanus toxin (Ross & Lawhorn, 1990). The single-fibre EMG has been used to detect the blockage of neuromuscular transmissions induced by organophosphates. This is a more sensitive measure than the EMG with repetitive nerve stimulation (Yang et al., 1996).

5.2.3.6 Spinal reflex excitability

Segmental spinal monosynaptic and polysynaptic reflexes are relatively simple functions in the CNS that can be evaluated by quantitative techniques (IPCS, 1986b). Many of the procedures used in animals are similar to procedures used clinically to perform neurological tests in humans. One approach infers the functional state of a reflex arc either from the latency and magnitude of the reflex response evoked by stimuli of predetermined intensity or from the stimulus intensity required to elicit a detectable response (i.e., the threshold). This approach is used best in a screening context, and the significance of effects in this test should be considered on a case-by-case basis.

A second, more involved approach records electrophysiologically the time required for a stimulus applied to a peripheral nerve to reach the spinal cord and return to the site of the original stimulation. Data from this procedure can indicate the excitability of the motoneuron pool, an effect seen with many volatile solvents. Although this approach is more invasive and time-consuming than the non-invasive procedure, it provides better data concerning the possible site of action (Wright et al., 1988). In addition, the manner in which the invasive procedure is carried out (e.g., in decerebrated animals) may preclude repeated testing on the same animal. The significance of effects in this procedure should also be considered on a case-by-case basis.

1.2.3.7   Ion channel function and synaptic transmission

Electrophysiological techniques, such as intracellular micro-electrode recording, iontophoresis, and voltage or patch clamp, enable cellular mechanisms of action of neurotoxicants to be determined (Audesirk, 1995; Shafer & Atchison, 1995). The electrical activity and metabolism of neurons are regulated by voltage-sensitive and ligand-sensitive mechanisms. Voltage-sensitive sodium, calcium and potassium channels are the most thoroughly studied voltage-sensitive channels. Ligand-sensitive mechanisms include many plasma membrane receptors and other receptors associated with G-proteins. Such procedures are not used routinely for screening except for certain compounds known to affect specific channels. At the sodium channel, for example, toxins can act through blockade (tetrodotoxin), activation (batrachotoxin) or a change in voltage sensitivity/activation (DDT) of channels (Shafer, 1999).

1.2.3.8   Hippocampal field potentials

The hippocampus is a region in the brain that has demonstrated potential for synaptic plasticity following activation (Gilbert & Burdette, 1995). One physiologically important change in the hippocampus is long-term potentiation (LTP), which may be defined as a persistent activity-dependent increase in the strength of synaptic transmission. It has been argued that the mechanisms underlying the development of LTP are similar to those supporting some forms of learning and memory. LTP can be studied *in vivo* and *in vitro* and has been shown to be affected by several neurotoxic chemicals, including chlorinated hydrocarbons, formamidines, pyrethroids, trimethyltin, lead, methylmercury and aluminium. Progress in this area may aid understanding of subtle changes in brain function that are associated with repeated, low-level exposure to neurotoxic agents.

5.2.4 Neurochemical end-points

Many different neurochemical end-points have been measured in neurotoxicological studies, and some have proven useful in advancing the understanding of mechanisms of action of neurotoxic chemicals (Bondy, 1986; Mailman, 1987; Morell & Mailman, 1987; Silbergeld, 1987; Costa, 1988; Ali & Slikker, 1995; Manzo et al., 1996). Functioning of the nervous system depends on the synthesis and release of specific neurotransmitters and activation of their receptors at specific pre-synaptic and post-synaptic sites (Ladefoged et al., 1995). Chemicals can interfere with the ionic balance of a neuron, act as a cytotoxicant after transport into a nerve terminal, block reuptake of neurotransmitters and their precursors, act as a metabolic poison, overstimulate receptors, block transmitter release and inhibit transmitter synthetic or catabolic enzymes. Table 12 lists several chemicals that produce neurotoxic effects at the neurochemical level (Bondy, 1986; Mailman, 1987; Morell & Mailman, 1987; Costa, 1988; Ali & Slikker, 1995).

Table 12. Known neurochemical modes of action of neurotoxicants in animals

Site of action	Examples
Neurotoxicants acting on ionic balance:	
A. Inhibit sodium entry	Tetrodotoxin
B. Delay closing of sodium channel	p,p'-DDT, pyrethroids
C. Increase permeability to sodium	Batrachotoxin
D. Increase intracellular calcium	Chlordecone, methylmercury
Uptake blockers	Hemicholinium
Block of respiratory function	Cyanide, MPTP
Hyperactivation of receptors	Domoic acid
Blocks transmitter release	Botulinum toxin
Inhibition of transmitter degradation	Organophosphate and carbamate pesticides
Increased neurotransmitter release	Tridimefon
Inhibition of succinic dehydrogenase	3-Nitropropionate

Any chemical-induced neurochemical change could be potentially neurotoxic (Ladefoged et al., 1995). For purposes of risk assessment, persistent or irreversible chemically induced neurochemical changes should be viewed with a high degree of concern. Because the ultimate functional significance of some biochemical changes is not known at this time, neurochemical studies should be interpreted with reference to the presumed neurotoxic consequences of the neurochemical changes (ECETOC, 1992). For example, many neuroactive agents can increase or decrease neurotransmitter levels, but such changes are not indicative of a neurotoxic effect. If, however, these neurochemical changes may be expected to have neurophysiological, neuropathological or neurobehavioural correlates, then the neurochemical changes could be classified as neurotoxic effects.

2.4.1   General biochemical measures

General biochemical end-points can be used to determine the integrity of nerve cells. Such general biochemical measures include end-points of cellular toxicity, changes in energy-linked functions or changes in synthesis of cell constituents or proteins. For end-points related to cell death, generally accepted criteria for adverse effects exist, whereas for other end-points, criteria may be problematic and should be correlated with other neurotoxic end-points. Changes in myelin basic protein indicative of alterations in lipid composition of the nerve can reflect demyelination (Norton & Cammer, 1984; Manzo et al., 1996). Changes in myelin basic protein may be determined to quantify myelination in the brain or reactive synthesis secondary to toxic insult. Heat shock proteins (HSP) are synthesized in cells in response to a variety of stresses, including exposure to neurotoxic compounds (Gonzalez et al., 1989). When the mechanism of neurotoxicity is known and a relevant biochemical end-point can be defined, direct measurement of this end-point may provide a sensitive estimate of neurotoxicity. Decreases in mRNA or protein synthesis, increased production of oxygen radicals (LeBel et al., 1990; Bondy, 1997) or changes in energy-related functions (Lai et al., 1980) may provide evidence for a neurotoxic effect (ECETOC, 1992).

5.2.4.2   Cholinesterase-inhibiting compounds

Some neurotoxicants, such as the organophosphate and carbamate pesticides, are known to inhibit the activity of a specific enzyme, AChE (Costa, 1988), which hydrolyses the neurotransmitter acetylcholine. Inhibition of the enzyme in either the CNS or PNS prolongs the action of the acetylcholine at the neuron's synaptic receptors and is thought to be responsible for the range of effects that these chemicals produce.

There is agreement that objective clinical measures of cholinergic overstimulation (e.g., salivation, sweating, muscle weakness, tremor, blurred vision) can be used to evaluate dose–response and dose–effect relationships and define the presence and absence of effects. A given depression in red cell, plasma or brain AChE activity may or may not be accompanied by clinical manifestations, depending on its magnitude and time course. Inhibition of red blood cell or plasma cholinesterase activity is a biomarker of exposure (Maxwell et al., 1987; ECETOC, 1992; Padilla et al., 1994; US EPA, 1998a).

Tolerance to the cholinergic overstimulation may be observed following repeated exposure to cholinesterase-inhibiting chemicals. It has been reported, however, that although tolerance can develop to some effects of cholinesterase inhibition, the cellular mechanisms responsible for the development of tolerance may also lead to the development of other effects, i.e., cognitive dysfunction, not present at the time of initial exposure (Bushnell et al., 1991).

In general, the assessment of cholinesterase-inhibiting chemicals should be done on a case-by-case basis using a weight-of-evidence approach in which all of the available data (e.g., brain, blood and other tissue cholinesterase activity, as well as the presence or absence of clinical signs) are considered in the evaluation. Generally, the acute cholinergic effects of anticholinesterase compounds are viewed as reversible (ECETOC, 1998), although longer-lasting effects have been reported in animals (Tandon et al., 1994). There is no experimental evidence for lasting or persistent effects of repeated exposure to organophosphates at levels that are not acutely toxic (Ray, 1999a).

A subset of organophosphate agents also produces organo-phosphate-induced delayed neuropathy (OPIDN) after acute or repeated exposure. This is characterized by degeneration of long axons in both peripheral nerves and the spinal cord. Inhibition and aging of neuropathy target enzyme (NTE) are associated with the initiation of OPIDN (Johnson, 1990; Richardson, 1995). Comparisons between the semi-log relationship between dose and NTE inhibition and the clinical outcome indicate that OPIDN develops when more than 70% of NTE inhibition/aging has occurred. This suggests that a certain degree of NTE inhibition, although not correlated with clinical neuropathy, represents the potential to cause OPIDN.

2.4.3 Cellular protein markers

The area of neurotoxicology that currently lags behind other areas of toxicology is the development of biomarkers (Costa, 1996). Some of this lack of progress can be attributed to the complexity of the nervous system and the multiplicity of the expression of the neurotoxic effects, along with the limited information on the mechanism of action at the target sites. Currently, the most developed approach using biomarkers is that with markers of exposure. Examples are the measurements of neurotoxic chemicals and metabolites in biological fluids, haemoglobin or albumin adducts, or metabolic enzymes. Progress has been slow in the development of biomarkers of effect because of the diversity in the mechanism of action and target sites involved in neurotoxic effects. Thus, the development of generic markers for neurotoxicity is not likely to be feasible. It appears that the development of biomarkers for a specific class of compounds or a specific target process is more reasonable. A number of proteins can be used to monitor the reactive changes seen in response to neuro-toxicity (Eng, 1988). Thus, the upregulation of lysosomal enzymes, the induction of early response genes or the production of cytokines can be used as biomarkers. However, before these can be used for risk assessment, questions of specificity and sensitivity need to be addressed. In addition, many potential biomarkers may show changes only over a relatively limited time window.

One of the better characterized biomarkers is glial fibrillary acidic protein (GFAP), the major intermediate filament protein in astrocytes (Amaducci et al., 1981). Although variably expressed by normal astrocytes, this cytoskeletal protein is markedly upregulated during reactive hypertrophy. In some cases, these astrocytic changes can be seen light microscopically with immunohistochemical stains for GFAP. In addition, GFAP can be quantified by an immunoassay, which has been proposed for use as a marker of astrocyte reactivity (O'Callaghan, 1988). Immunohistochemical stains have the advantage of better localization of GFAP increases, whereas immunoassay evaluations are superior at quantifying changes in GFAP levels and establishing dose–response relationships (Bignami & Dahl, 1976). The ability to detect and quantify changes in GFAP by immunoassay is improved by dissecting and analysing multiple brain regions. The interpretation of a chemical-induced change in GFAP is greatly facilitated by corroborative data from the neuropathology or neuro-anatomy evaluation. A number of chemicals known to injure the CNS, including trimethyltin, methylmercury, cadmium, 3-acetylpyridine and MPTP, have been shown to increase levels of GFAP.

Increases in GFAP above control levels may be seen at dosages below those necessary to produce damage seen by non-immuno-histochemical microscopic or histopathological techniques. Because increases in GFAP reflect an astrocyte response in adults, treatment-related increases in GFAP are considered to be evidence that a cellular reaction that reflects a neurotoxic effect has occurred (O'Callaghan, 1988). There is less agreement as to how to interpret decreases in GFAP relative to an appropriate control group. The absence of a change in GFAP following exposure does not mean that the chemical is devoid of neurotoxic potential. Known neurotoxicants with a pharmacological mode of action, such as cholinesterase-inhibiting pesticides, would not be expected to increase brain levels of GFAP. Interpretation of GFAP changes prior to weaning may be confounded by the possibility that chemically induced increases in GFAP could be masked by changes in the concentration of this protein associated with maturation of the CNS, and these data may be difficult to interpret. Chemical-induced changes in GFAP may be transient and could be missed if measured outside of the relevant time window.

5.2.5 Neuroendocrine end-points

Many types of behaviours (e.g., reproductive behaviours, sexual behaviours) are dependent on the integrity of the hypothalamic–

pituitary system, which could represent an important site for neurotoxic action (US NRC, 1992; Tilson, 1998b; Weiss, 1998). Pituitary secretions arise from a number of different cell types in this gland, and neurotoxicants could affect these cells either directly or indirectly. Morphological changes in follicular cells, chromophobe cells, somatotrophic cells, prolactin cells, gonadotrophic cells, follicle stimulating hormone secreting cells, luteinizing hormone containing cells and thyrotrophic cells might be associated with adverse effects on the pituitary, which could ultimately affect behaviour and the functioning of the nervous system.

Biochemical changes in the hypothalamus may also be used as indices of potential changes in neuroendocrine function. However, the neuroendocrine significance of changes in hypothalamic neurotransmitters and neuropeptides is usually only inferential, and data must be considered on a case-by-case basis.

Most anterior pituitary hormones are subject to negative feedback control by peripheral endocrine glands, and, if neurotoxicants modify peripheral secretions, neuroendocrine changes can result from this altered feedback. Modifications in the functioning of these endocrine secretions could occur after toxic exposure; a number of agents have been shown to alter blood levels of glucocorticoids, thyroxine, estrogen, corticosterone and testosterone. Although such changes are not necessarily due to direct neuroendocrine effects, target organ changes can often be a first indication of neuroendocrine changes. Chemically induced changes in hormonal levels are logically linked to histopathological changes in target neuroendocrine sites. Stress resulting from experimental manipulation of the animal by dosing or test procedures must be taken into account in the interpretation of changes in neuroendocrine function.

5.2.6 Structural end-points

Methods to measure chemical-induced neurotoxicity have been reviewed in detail elsewhere (IPCS, 1986b; ECETOC, 1992), and this document will provide general background information and focus on recent developments. McMartin et al. (1997) published a simplified nomenclature for non-proliferative pathological changes occurring in the rat nervous system based primarily on histopathological findings in haematoxylin- and eosin-stained tissue. Techniques of value in neuropathology have also been reviewed by Chang (1995). Quantitative morphometric techniques have been reviewed by Scallet (1995). Structural end-points are typically defined as neuropathological changes evident by gross observation or light microscopy, although most neurotoxic changes will not be readily detected at the gross observational level and require more detailed examination.

A significant dose-dependent decrease in brain weight is generally considered to be a biologically significant effect. This is usually true regardless of changes in body weight, because brain weight is generally assumed to be spared under conditions of mild undernutrition. It is generally inappropriate to express brain weight changes as a ratio of body weight and thereby dismiss changes in absolute brain weight. Given the paucity of historical data in the toxicology literature on changes in length or width of brain, fresh brain weight is considered to be a more reliable indicator of alteration in brain structure. Other gross changes include brain swelling as a result of oedema or vacuolation of the neuropil. Subdural or petechial haemorrhages can also be observed on exposing or cutting down the tissue.

Various types of neuropathological lesions may be classified according to the site where they occur (Spencer & Schaumburg, 1980; IPCS, 1986b; Krinke, 1989; Griffin, 1990). Standardized nomenclature should be used (McMartin et al., 1997). Neurotoxicant-induced lesions in the CNS or PNS may be classified as a neuronopathy (changes in the neuronal cell body), axonopathy (changes in the axons), myelinopathy (changes in the myelin sheaths) or nerve terminal degeneration. Non-neuronal cells may also be targeted by neurotoxicants, notably oligodendrocytes and Schwann cells (cuprizone), astrocytes (α-chlorohydrin) and endothelial cells (dinitrobenzene) (Romero et al., 1991). Some agents (e.g., nitropropionate) can target neurons, glia and blood vessels (Ray, 1999b).

Within each general class of nervous system structural alteration, there are various histological changes that can result after exposure to neurotoxicants. The degenerative process of the nerve cell can be either a relatively rapid or prolonged process depending on the underlying mechanism responsible. The reactions of neurons to injury vary dramatically. Neurons can degenerate following a direct action on the cell body or following loss of synaptic target site influences or trophic factors. Various types of neuronal response include the accumulation, proliferation or rearrangement of structural elements or organelles. Some classifications generally used in evaluating neuronal degeneration include central chromatolysis, where Nissl granules disappear around a swollen eccentric nucleus, peripheral chromatolysis, as defined by lack of Nissl substance near the cell membrane, and simple chromatolysis, where there is a diffuse loss of Nissl granules with swollen cytoplasm and axons. Other severe changes associated with neuronal degeneration can include a cell nucleus that is hyperchromatic, shrunken and pyknotic with swollen eosinophilic cytoplasm. Ischaemic changes in the neuron are characterized by a loss of affinity for stains and by nuclear changes (e.g., elongation, chromatin clumps, disappearance of nuclear membrane). These changes are usually irreversible. A common chronic response of the neuron is a shrinkage of the cell body and nucleus. The intact internal structures are crowded, and the cell border takes on a triangular shape. Neurons may survive in this state for an extended period of time; however, the changes are usually irreversible and eventually lead to cell sclerosis, where the cell constituents clump or disintegrate.

Dying neurons can autophagocytize or undergo apoptosis with a condensation and dissolution of chromatin and transfer of chromatin into cytoplasmic autophagocytic vacuoles (Clarke & Hornung, 1989). Neuronal death may also be caused by failure to obtain critical amounts of neurotrophic factors and the proper retrograde transport of such factors.

The majority of research regarding toxicant-induced damage to axons has been conducted in the PNS. In this system, axonopathies have been characterized by location of damage, i.e., proximal or distal region of the axon. Proximal refers to the area of transition from the cell body to the axon (axon hillock) and the proximal portion of the axon. The proximal axon is selectively involved in relatively few cases. One of the major changes is the formation of giant axonal swellings containing 10-nm neurofilaments following β,β'-iminodipropionitrile intoxication and in motor neuron degeneration, including human ALS and hereditary canine spinal muscular atrophy (Ferri et al., 1994). The majority of axonopathic chemicals produce perturbations in the distal portions of the axon, which, for hexacarbon (e.g., *n*-hexane) and carbon disulfide intoxication, can display giant axonal swellings similar to those found in proximal axonopathies. These swellings begin multifocally in the preterminal regions of axons and progress to more proximal regions with continued exposure. It has been proposed that such axonopathies are associated with neurofilamentous accumulations; however, such accumulations of neurofilaments are often a more late stage event, as is the case for acrylamide, suggesting an associated but not a causal relationship. Although nerve terminal degeneration may occur, it represents a very subtle change that may not be detected by routine histopathology, but requires detection by special procedures such as silver staining or neurotransmitter-specific immunohistochemistry. Functionally, such degeneration may be evident in the PNS as muscle atrophy due to lack of appropriate neural innervation.

The myelin membrane is highly vulnerable to damage from exposure to toxic substances, which can result in the loss of the myelin sheath (demyelination) or in alterations in the myelin sheath without producing actual demyelination (dysmyelination). Demyelination can occur following a direct perturbation to the myelinating cell or its myelin sheath or as a response to axonal degeneration. In the PNS, the process of demyelination is a sequence of the Schwann cell differentiating to autophagocytize its own plasmalemma, proliferating and remyelinating the damaged region of the axon with smaller internodes. Often the only way to detect a demyelinating disorder is to observe evidence of remyelination. Dysmyelination, however, can include folding and oedematous splitting at various levels of the myelin lamella.

The nervous system is dependent on an extensive system of blood vessels and capillaries to deliver large quantities of oxygen and nutrients, as well as to remove toxic waste products. Damage to the capillaries in the brain can lead to a swelling characteristic of encephalopathy. Vascular damage may be important in the pathogenesis of neurotoxicity, but can be hard to detect and evaluate in the absence of gross changes unless specialized methods are used. Vascular breakdown and astrocytic involvement were prominent features of the 3-nitropropionic acid lesions described by Nishino et al. (1997); however, many other studies that did not use immunohistochemical methods to visualize leakage of plasma protein did not report vascular damage. Other studies of this and other agents have failed to report damage due to the use of insufficiently short survival times (Ray, 1997). If a recovery period of more than a week is allowed, mild vascular damage will resolve, and serious vascular damage will develop into an infarct in which primary and secondary damage become indistinguishable. Visualization of vascular damage is aided by the use of thick sections and by staining for leakage of natural or artificial intravascular markers, such as albumin or fluorophores. Haemorrhagic lesions of the nervous system have been noted in the brains or PNS of rats exposed to cadmium during development or as adults (Gabbiani et al., 1967; Klaassen, 1982; Murthy et al., 1987).

Virtually every class of injury that alters CNS function is associated with a neuroglial response (Eng, 1988; Yu et al., 1993). This gliotic activation can be associated with sublethal insults to neurons and may contribute to their survival (Cavanagh et al., 1990). In relatively mild injury, the astrocytic properties supporting homeostasis can also serve to restore order. Injury sufficient to kill neurons is usually accompanied by a reactive change in astrocyte structure and function. Reactive astrocytes (astrogliosis) display hypertrophy, extend thick, long processes, elevate glutamine synthetase and oxido-reductive enzyme activity, and significantly increase their cytoplasmic content of GFAP (Eng, 1985, 1988). The gliotic response is a dynamic process that is regionally specific. However, it is often wider than the injury itself, and the nature of the lesion can change significantly with time. While increased mRNA or protein content for GFAP can be detected soon after an injury to the CNS, these are relatively late-occurring changes. By the time that an increase in astroglial changes is detectable, signals have likely already been given to the astrocytes. A possible cellular source for this rapid signal is the microglia.

Microglial cells have been demonstrated to respond rapidly to even minor pathological changes in the CNS (Streit et al., 1988; Giulian et al., 1989; Dickson et al., 1991; Perry et al., 1993; Gehrmann et al., 1995; Gebicke-Haerter et al., 1996; Kreutzberg, 1996). The activation of microglia can serve as a major factor in the defence of the neural parenchyma against a number of insults, including infectious diseases, inflammation, trauma, ischaemia, tumors and neurodegeneration. Injury-activated microglia are characterized by hypertrophy, proliferation, increased surface expression of immune marker molecules, increased migration, release of oxygen radicals and proteases, and differentiation into a macrophage-like phenotype (Banati et al., 1993; Giulian et al., 1994). Such responses may be beneficial in the healing phases of CNS injury by actively monitoring and controlling the extracellular environment, walling off areas of the CNS from non-CNS tissue and removing dead or damaged cells (Giulian et al., 1989; Banati et al., 1993; Yu et al., 1993). This gliotic process, however, is also thought to impart detrimental consequences by collateral neuronal damage from released microglial cytotoxins and inhibit neuronal regeneration by physical or biochemical impediments.

Table 13 (IPCS, 1986b) lists examples of neurotoxic chemicals, their putative site of action, the type of neuropathology produced and the disorder or condition that each typifies. Inclusion of any chemical in the table is for illustrative purposes only — i.e., it has been reported that the chemical will produce a neurotoxic effect at some dose; any individual chemical listed may also adversely affect other organs at lower doses.

Alterations in the structure of the nervous system (i.e., neuronopathy, axonopathy, myelinopathy, terminal degeneration) are regarded as evidence of a neurotoxic effect. The risk assessor should note that pathological changes in many cases require time for the perturbation to become observable, especially with evaluation at the light microscopic level. Neuropathological studies should control for potential differences in the areas and sections of the nervous system sampled or omitted, in the age, sex and body weight of the subject, and in fixation artefacts (IPCS, 1986b). Concern for the structural integrity of nervous system tissues derives from its functional specialization and the limited regenerative capacity in the CNS.

The nervous system presents numerous specific challenges to structural investigation. These are due to its macroscopic complexity and diversity, which cause major difficulties in tissue sampling. In order to achieve a reasonably comprehensive survey of the CNS, representative coronal sections need to be examined from multiple levels. Many guidelines for such sectioning have determined that this requires at least five levels, as detailed in IPCS (1986b). Otherwise, it is entirely possible to miss significant focal lesions. The susceptibility of the brain to anoxic insult and to excitotoxicity makes it very

Table 13. Examples of toxic effects and patterns of structural damage in
laboratory animals

Pattern	Cause
Neuronal changes	
Laminar cortical necrosis	Anoxia
Hippocampal pyramidal cell damage (rat) Hippocampal dentate granule cell damage (rat, mouse)	Trimethyltin
Purkinje cell loss (cerebellum)	Penitrem, methylmercury
Loss of inferior olivary cells	3-Acetylpyridine
Degeneration of perikarya of sensory ganglion cells	Doxorubicin
Degeneration of axons of sensory ganglion cells; optic area of cortex	Methylmercury
Degeneration of long sensory or motor axons in CNS and PNS	Organophosphates, acrylamide, 2,5-hexane-dione, carbon disulfide
Necrosis of striatum	3-Nitropropionic acid
Degeneration of optic nerve	Clioquinol
Myelin changes	
CNS myelin vacuolation	Triethyltin
CNS and PNS myelin vacuolation	Hexachlorophene
Focal degeneration of PNS myelin without axon loss	Diphtheria, lead
Focal degeneration of PNS myelin with some axon loss	Lead
Vascular and necrotic changes	
Symmetrical changes in brainstem nuclei	Dinitrobenzene
Non-symmetrical brainstem and cortical lesions	Lead

vulnerable to postmortem artefact (e.g., shrunken dense neurons). This can be minimized by arterial perfusion with fixative under terminal anaesthesia. Where this is not practicable, great care has to be taken to distinguish postmortem damage from in-life damage. The most useful indicators of postmortem damage are a lack of a dose–response relationship and the lack of a tissue reaction, such as an increase in the glial response. Routine preparations of peripheral nerve are also susceptible to a postmortem artefact, and, where peripheral nerve damage is suspected, teased fibre preparations can be an invaluable aid to interpretation (King, 1999). In both the CNS and the PNS, examination of the myelin sheath is plagued with artefact, due to both postmortem damage and poor perfusion fixation. These artefacts are even more pronounced when myelin is examined at the electron microscopic level.

New or improved histological stains and antibodies are now available to detect and characterize effects of neurotoxicants. For example, silver impregnation stains for degenerating axons were, for many years, used primarily by neuroanatomists to trace degenerating nerve tracts in the CNS after experimental lesions. Early versions of this staining procedure were cumbersome to use, and results were often capricious. However, recent developments in sectioning and staining technology now allow this technique to be used more efficiently to demonstrate neurotoxicant-induced lesions (Switzer, 2000). Silver impregnation stains sometimes reveal more neuronal damage than traditional Nissl or H&E stains (Balaban et al., 1988) and enable traditional light microscopic examination to detect lesions in structures (e.g., nerve terminals, unmyelinated axons) otherwise visible only by electron microscopy (Ritter & Dinh, 1988). Fluoro-Jade has shown similar promise as a fluorescent marker of damage (Schmued & Hopkins, 2000). Terminal deoxynucleotidyl transferase-mediated deoxyuridine triphosphate nick-end labelling stains may be used to determine apoptotic neurodegeneration (Ikonomidou et al., 2000); however, additional morphological evaluation may be required, as this staining may also pick out cells dying by necrosis.

A wide variety of immunohistochemical markers are also available for all major cell types, for intracellular structures and for major neurotransmitter systems (Table 14). As a result, light microscopy can now be used to detect and characterize neurotoxicant-induced changes that previously (IPCS, 1986b) required regional chemical assays or electron microscopy. For example, changes in serotonin immunoreactivity in the dorsal and median raphe nuclei of rats have been demonstrated in the offspring of rats whose dams were exposed to 2,4-dichlorophenoxyacetic acid throughout lactation (Evangelista de Duffard et al., 1995b). With the exception of the extensive database for

Table 14. Examples of immunohistochemical markers of particular value for neurotoxicological evaluations

Tissue	Antibodies	Comment
Neuronal cell body	Neurofilament proteins Calbindin 28K NeuN	These normal cellular constituents are altered in a variety of neurological disease states
Astrocytes	GFAP	Hypertrophic astrocytes may be common response to injury in CNS
Microglia	ED-1, OX-42, B$_4$ lectin	Microglia activation may be common response to injury in CNS
Neurons and glia	β-amyloid precursor protein	May be increased in a variety of CNS disease states
Vasculature	IgG	Leakage of plasma protein can indicate damage to BBB
All cell types	HSP and ubiquitin	Changes in HSP and ubiquitin may indicate early cellular response to insult

the astrocyte-specific marker GFAP, the use of these antibodies in the area of neurotoxicology has yet to be validated.

5.2.7   Axonal transport

Axonal transport represents a process that is critical to the functioning and maintenance of the neuronal processes and thus may be a critical target site of toxic chemicals (Sabri, 1986; Ochs, 1987). A number of toxicants produce morphological alterations in the axons of peripheral nerves and alterations in axonal transport. Transport may be altered in a number of different ways: (1) an agent may interact with a specific step in the mechanism of axonal transport; (2) the movement of a specific transported component may be altered; or (3) a general biochemical process, such as energy metabolism, may be perturbed. An alteration in a general biochemical process such as the disruption of energy metabolism has been proposed as an underlying mechanism altering axonal transport and producing distal axonopathy (Spencer et al., 1979, 1987a; Brimijoin & Hammond, 1985). Structural components intrinsic to the axonal transport system are a point of vulnerability and may be directly altered.

Distal axonal swellings, composed of accumulations of smooth endoplasmic reticulum-derived vesiculotubular membrane structures, are produced by several neurotoxic chemicals, including *p*-bromophenylacetylurea, zinc pyridine thione and certain organophosphorus compounds (for review, see Harry, 1999). It is unknown whether the changes reflect a direct effect of the toxicant on smooth endoplasmic reticulum or a non-specific reactive response of the axon. While slow axonal transport is the main transport component that is altered with accumulations of neurofilaments, chemicals that produce accumulations of membranous structures appear to have little or no effect on slow axonal transport until the axonopathy is severe and the axon shows signs of degeneration.

Some toxicants produce a primary alteration in the cell body rather than the axon. Although the primary site of morphological perturbation is the cell body, alterations in axonal transport can be seen as the result of alterations in the complex processes of transport initiation. Of the representative compounds proposed to produce a peripheral neuropathy by altering axonal transport, acrylamide is probably the most thoroughly studied (Harry, 1992; Harry et al., 1992). Following exposure to acrylamide, peripheral nerves display a multifocal distal axonopathy characterized by axonal swellings localized at the nodes of Ranvier and distal axonal degeneration.

Most studies that examine alterations in axonal transport rely on the use of whole animals; due to the complex nature of the process, *in vivo* studies will probably remain the major experimental system. *In vitro* techniques, such as the video-enhanced contrast differential interference contrast microscopy methodology, allow specific questions on organelle movement along the axon to be addressed. They have contributed to the identification and understanding of the molecular mechanisms and motors of transport, kinesis and dynein (Brady et al., 1985; Brady, 1991), but have been less successful in addressing general questions of toxicant-induced alterations of axonal transport and peripheral neuropathies (Brat & Brimijoin, 1993; Martenson et al., 1995; Sickles et al., 1996).

5.3   Special issues in developmental neurotoxicity

All of the neurotoxicity end-points discussed previously apply to studies in which either adult or developmental end-points are used. However, there are particular issues of importance in the evaluation of developmental animal neurotoxicity studies. This section underscores the importance of detecting neurotoxic effects following developmental exposure. In comparison with adults, data have indicated (US NRC, 1993) that infants and children may be differentially sensitive and differentially exposed to environmental chemicals such as pesticides. Exposure to chemicals during development can result in a spectrum of effects, including death, structural abnormalities, altered growth and functional deficits (IPCS, 1984; Slikker, 1997). A number of agents have been shown to cause developmental neurotoxicity when exposure occurred during the period between conception and sexual maturity (Riley & Vorhees, 1986; Vorhees, 1987; Kimmel & Kimmel, 1996; Tilson, 1998b; US NRC, 2000). Table 15 lists several examples of agents known to produce developmental neurotoxicity in experimental animals. Animal models of developmental neurotoxicity have been shown to be sensitive to several environmental agents known to produce developmental neurotoxicity in humans, including lead, ethanol, X-irradiation, methylmercury and PCBs (Jacobson et al., 1985; Needleman, 1987, 1990; Kimmel et al., 1990). In many of these cases, functional deficits are observed at dose levels below those at which other indicators of developmental toxicity are evident or at minimally toxic doses in adults. In other cases, the effects are primarily morphological, such as the disruption of the normal segmental development of the brain produced by embryonic exposure to valproate, which results in spina bifida or brainstem abnormalities (Bojic et al., 1998). Developmental exposure to a chemical could result in transient or apparently reversible effects observed early during development that could re-emerge as the individual ages (Reuhl, 1991; Barone et al., 1995).

Important design issues to be evaluated for developmental neuro-toxicity studies are similar to those for standard developmental toxicity studies, such as (1) use of a dose–response approach, with the highest dose producing minimal overt maternal or perinatal toxicity; (2) use of a large enough number of litters for adequate statistical power; (3) randomization of animals to dose groups and test groups; and (4) consideration of the litter as the statistical unit. In some cases, particularly in order to control for postnatal maternal effects on offspring or

Table 15. Examples of compounds producing developmental neurotoxicity in humans and animal models

Class of compounds	Examples
Alcohols	Methanol, ethanol
Antimitotics	Azacytidine
Insecticides	DDT, chlordecone
Metals	Lead, methylmercury, cadmium
Anticonvulsants	Valproate, phenytoin
Polyhalogenated hydrocarbons	PCBs, PBBs

to precisely define periods of differential vulnerability, it is desirable to separate the influence of pre- and postnatal factors. In such cases, pups, once born, may be distributed to other dams in a procedure known as cross-fostering (Nelson, 1986). Depending on the specific testing protocol used, exposure may occur during narrow time frames in gestation or lactation or within defined developmental periods, such as prenatal, preweaning, postweaning or any combination of these. In order to separate effects of prenatal exposure on brain development and associated behavioural disruption from effects mediated through altered maternal behaviour postnatally, it may be necessary to introduce cross-fostering procedures into the study design. For example, the prenatal origin of persistent PCB-induced behavioural alterations has been shown in rats by Lilienthal & Winneke (1991). In studies utilizing cross-fostering, the postnatal environment of all animals should be similar, animals should be tested concurrently and litters should be culled to a common number and gender of offspring by postnatal day 2 (Nelson, 1986). In addition, the use of a replicate study design provides added confidence in the interpretation of data.

Direct extrapolation of developmental neurotoxicity to humans is limited in the same way as for other end-points of toxicity, i.e., by the lack of knowledge about underlying toxicological mechanisms and their significance (Cory-Slechta, 1990; US EPA, 1991b). Known cross-species differences in nervous system development should be taken into account. Comparisons of human and animal data for several agents known to cause developmental neurotoxicity in humans showed many similarities in effects (Kimmel et al., 1990). As evidenced primarily by observations in laboratory animals, comparisons at the level of functional category (sensory, motivational, cognitive and motor function and social behaviour) showed close agreement across species for the agents evaluated, even though the specific end-points used to assess these functions varied considerably across species (Stanton & Spear, 1990). Thus, it can be assumed that developmental neurotoxicity effects in animal studies indicate the potential for altered neurobehavioural development in humans, although the specific types of developmental effects seen in experimental animal studies will not be the same as those that may be produced in humans. Therefore, when data suggesting adverse effects in developmental neurotoxicity studies are encountered for particular agents, they should be considered in the risk assessment process. A series of tests conducted in animals in several age groups may provide more information about maturational changes and their persistence than tests conducted at a single age.

It is a well established principle that there are critical developmental periods for the disruption of functional competence, which include both the prenatal and postnatal periods to the time of sexual maturation, and the effect of a toxicant is likely to vary depending on the onset and duration of exposure relative to this development (Rodier, 1986, 1990). It is also important to consider the data from studies in which postnatal exposure is included, as there may be an interaction of the agent with maternal behaviour, milk composition and pup suckling behaviour, as well as possible direct exposure of pups via dosed food or water (Kimmel et al., 1992).

Agents that produce developmental neurotoxicity at a dose that is not toxic to the maternal animal are of special concern. However, adverse developmental effects are often produced at doses that cause mild maternal toxicity (e.g., 10–20% reduction in weight gain during gestation and lactation). At doses causing moderate maternal toxicity (i.e., 20% or more reduction in weight gain during gestation and lactation), interpretation of developmental effects may be confounded. Current information is inadequate to assume that developmental effects at doses causing minimal maternal toxicity result only from maternal toxicity; rather, it may be that the mother and developing organism are equally sensitive to that dose level. Moreover, whether developmental effects are secondary to maternal toxicity or not, the maternal effects may be reversible, while the effects on the offspring may be permanent. These are important considerations for agents to which humans may be exposed at maternally toxic levels.

Although interpretability of developmental neurotoxicity data may be limited, it is clear that functional effects must be evaluated in light of other toxicity data, including other forms of developmental toxicity (e.g., structural abnormalities, perinatal death, growth retardation). For example, alterations in motor performance may be due to a skeletal malformation rather than nervous system change. Changes in learning tasks that require a visual cue might be influenced by structural abnormalities in the eye. The level of confidence that an agent produces an adverse effect may be as important as the type of change seen, and confidence may be increased by such factors as reproducibility of the effect either in another study of the same function or by convergence of data from tests that purport to measure similar functions. A dose–response relationship is an extremely important measure of a chemical's effect; in the case of developmental neurotoxicity, both monotonic and biphasic dose–response curves are likely, depending on the function being tested.

Sometimes functional defects are observed at dose levels below those at which other indicators of developmental toxicity are evident (Rodier, 1986). Such effects may be transient or reversible in nature, but generally are considered adverse effects. Data from postnatal studies, when available, are considered useful for further assessment of the relative importance and severity of findings in the fetus and neonate. Often, the long-term consequences of adverse developmental outcomes noted at birth are unknown, and further data on postnatal development and function are necessary to determine the full spectrum of potential developmental effects. Useful data can also be derived from well conducted multigeneration studies, although the dose levels used in these studies may be much lower than those in studies with shorter-term exposure.

Much of the early work in developmental neurotoxicology was related to behavioural evaluations. Advances in this area have been reviewed in several publications (e.g., Kimmel & Kimmel, 1996; US NRC, 2000). Several expert groups have focused on the functions that should be included in a behavioural testing battery, including sensory systems, neuromotor development, locomotor activity, learning and memory, reactivity and habituation, and reproductive behaviour.

Direct extrapolation of functional developmental effects to humans is limited in the same way as for other end-points of developmental toxicity, i.e., by the lack of knowledge about underlying toxicological mechanisms and their significance. It can be assumed that functional effects in animal studies indicate the potential for altered development in humans, although the types of developmental effects seen in experimental animal studies will not necessarily be the same as those that may be produced in humans. Thus, when data from functional developmental toxicity studies are encountered for particular agents, they should be considered in the risk assessment process.

5.4   *In vitro* methods

Methods and procedures that fall under the general heading of short-term tests include an array of *in vitro* tests that have been proposed as alternatives to whole-animal tests (Goldberg & Frazier, 1989; Stokes & Marafante, 1998). In the field of neurobiology, *in vitro* cell culture techniques have been successfully developed and employed to address specific questions of cell biology and nervous system functioning. Cell culture techniques provide a means of systematically studying complex nervous systems (Arenander & deVellis, 1983; Fedoroff & Vernadakis, 1987; Saneto & deVellis, 1987; Shahar et al., 1989; Jacobson, 1991; Harry et al., 1998; Pentreath, 1999). In neurotoxicology, *in vitro* methods are not ordinarily considered as alternatives to *in vivo* procedures using the whole animal. Instead, *in vitro* methods are selected to address specific hypotheses. Studies with tissues, cells or cell fragments simply provide the most appropriate approach and, in many cases, could not be conducted in live animals. *In vitro* models are therefore used in an attempt to study biological processes in a more isolated context. They are most useful when a direct investigation of biological processes is difficult or impossible because of the complexity of the processes involved. *In vitro* models may also be appropriate whenever an experiment cannot be performed for ethical reasons. It is generally recognized that *in vitro* systems often provide only partial answers to more complex problems; therefore, they can supplement, but rarely replace, investigations with whole animals (Harry et al., 1998).

For many questions in biology and medicine, *in vitro* techniques may not be suitable. For example, *in vitro* techniques offer little information about a chemical effect on sensory or cognitive functions, but one can examine isolated actions taking place in receptor cells at the cellular and molecular level. If one is interested in investigating the effects on the central processing of the message received by the receptor cells, storage of this information in short- and long-term memory, or the behavioural and somatic responses resulting from some of the sensory perception, assessment of the whole animal is essential.

Various types of *in vitro* approaches produce data for evaluating potential and known neurotoxic substances, including primary cell cultures, cell lines and cloned cells. While such procedures are important in studying the mechanism of action of toxic agents, their use in screening chemicals for potential neurotoxicity in humans has not been widely established. Characteristics of an adequate screen for neurotoxic chemicals and estimation of neurotoxicological risk have been described (Walum et al., 1993). The use of *in vitro* tests for screening will require defined end-points of toxicity and understanding of how a test chemical would be handled *in vitro* compared with the intact organism. There is general agreement that *in vitro* data could be used to enhance the interpretation of *in vivo* data.

The physicochemical environment of cells is easily manipulated *in vitro* such that substances can be added or withdrawn from the culture medium, allowing precise temporal analysis of the sequences of events as they occur. On the other hand, the extrapolation of such data to the human is often difficult or impossible. Compounds that are insoluble either in aqueous systems or at neutral pH pose the problem that any artificial carrier or vehicle may be intrinsically toxic or may change the toxicological characteristics of the compounds. In cell cultures, a test compound that is not, or is only slowly, metabolized only allows for the intrinsic toxicity of a compound to be evaluated, so *in vitro* data from compounds that require metabolic activation, are quickly metabolized to non-toxic substances or fail to cross the BBB may not reflect the *in vivo* situation. Simulation of compound metabolism by the addition of microsomal additives or metabolically active cells is difficult to standardize or known to induce cytotoxicity. Local metabolic activation of some chemicals is crucial for their neurotoxic effect. Owing to limited survival of neural cells, many *in vitro* test systems do not allow for the prolonged exposure necessary for some neurotoxic effects to occur. The lack of regulatory control of neuroendocrine systems, nutritional support provided by the blood circulation, the BBB, which prohibits certain compounds from gaining access to the nervous system, and interaction with adjacent cells may hinder the extrapolation of *in vitro* results to *in vivo* situations. *In vitro* systems offer the opportunity to examine similar cell types from different species. The response of human cells can be compared with that of other species to address the question of interspecies selective toxicity. As primary cell cultures are not readily available from humans, experiments often use human cell lines. The response of cell lines may, however, be totally different from that of corresponding primary cell cultures and may change with continuous passages in culture. Primary cell cultures are enriched in any one particular cell type. Although such an isolated condition is an alien state for neural cells, it is also perceived as a major advantage to study a compound's effects on specific cell types. Furthermore, culture conditions used in *in vitro* preparations may markedly affect the outcome of the experiment.

Effects induced by a compound in an *in vitro* test system may be the result of cytotoxicity, a pharmacological effect of the compound or a neurotoxic effect. Differentiation between these three possible mechanisms is not always easy. One approach used to discriminate between neurotoxicity and general toxicity is to examine specific end-points unique to nervous system functions and to compare the dose–response relationships between neurotoxic end-points and end-points indicating general toxicity (Pentreath, 1999). Another approach is to compare toxic responses between neuronal and non-neuronal cells. Examples of basal cell functions used to differentiate between cytotoxicity and neurotoxicity are dye exclusion, DNA integrity, energy regulation, calcium homeostasis, biosynthetic reactions and indicators of mitochondrial and lysosomal activity.

Although often neglected, structural aspects can provide important information on the *in vitro* test system and its comparability to the *in vivo* situation. Morphological end-points include effects on the cell body, axons and dendrites. Neurons exposed to substances in culture often develop structurally abnormal neurites such as "beading," which indicates altered neurite outgrowth. Neuron-specific functions assessed as end-points of neurotoxicity encompass such diverse functions as axonal transport, receptor or ion channel expression and function, neurotransmitter synthesis and cell reactive changes. Many of these end-points are known to be affected by pharmaceutical agents. Therefore, for many of these end-points, it is difficult or impossible to set a criterion that allows one to differentiate between a pharmacological and a neurotoxic effect. For the process of risk assessment, such a discrimination is central. End-points used to determine potential neurotoxicity of a compound have to be carefully selected and evaluated with respect to their potential to discriminate between an adverse, neurotoxic effect and a pharmacological effect. It is obvious that for *in vitro* neurotoxicity studies, the primary end-points that can be used are those that are affected through specific mechanisms of neurotoxicity.

Due to the complexity of the nervous system, the multitude of functions of individual cells and our limited knowledge of the potential biochemical processes involved in neurotoxicity, it would be difficult to design an *in vitro* test battery that could replace *in vivo* test systems. *In vitro* tests have their greatest potential to be used — and today are most successfully used — to elucidate mechanisms of toxicity, identify target cells of neurotoxicity and delineate the development of intricate cellular changes induced by neurotoxicants. When *in vitro* test systems are used to screen for specific neurotoxic effects, end-points must be carefully selected to allow differentiation between cytotoxic, neurotoxic and pharmacological effects. For certain structurally defined compounds and mechanisms of toxicity, such as organophosphorus compounds and delayed neuropathy, for which target cells and the biochemical processes involved in the neurotoxicity are well known, an *in vitro* test system may be useful. For other compounds and the different types of neurotoxicity induced, biochemical end-points have to be identified that can be used in *in vitro* test systems to predict these types of neurotoxicity. Demonstrated neurotoxicity *in vitro* in the absence of *in vivo* data is suggestive but inadequate evidence of a neurotoxic effect. *In vivo* data supported by *in vitro* data enhance the reliability of the *in vivo* results.

5.5 Testing strategies for neurotoxicity

Standard toxicity studies generally include clinical observations, gross examination of most organs and tissues, measurement of the weight of organs, including the brain, and histopathological evaluation of many tissues (IPCS, 1986b; ECETOC, 1992; Ladefoged et al.,

1995). Information from such studies may give preliminary or definite indications of the neurotoxicity of chemicals. Specific testing protocols for neurotoxicity in adults and developing animals have been generated by intergovernmental organizations and national authorities, including the OECD, US EPA and US FDA (US EPA, 1991a; ECETOC, 1992; ICME, 1994; OECD, 1995, 1997, 1999; EC, 1996). Because of the large number of possible tests for neurotoxicity, tiered testing strategies have been developed (ECETOC, 1992; Johnsen et al., 1992). At the foundation of this approach are screening tests that are designed to detect potential neurotoxicity. Carefully conducted clinical observations or neurological assessments are used in conjunction with standard toxicity tests and are intended to provide significant information concerning possible neurotoxic effects. Based on such findings, additional end-points may be included to provide in-depth information about a specific type of neurotoxic effect. Additional research may also be conducted to further characterize the effects or mechanisms of known neurotoxicants.

In the European Union (EU), technical guidance for EU authorities has been provided (EC, 1996). It is recommended that a hierarchical approach be taken to assess the potential neurotoxicity of substances. Formal tier testing strategies are not routinely employed by regulatory agencies in the USA (Tilson et al., 1996). For example, for chemicals regulated under the US Federal Insecticide, Fungicide and Rodenticide Act, data from an established number of testing protocols are required for the registration and reregistration of pesticides. Based on several criteria, the Neurotoxicology Testing Battery or the Developmental Neurotoxicity Testing Guidelines may be requested from the US EPA, in addition to other required tests for carcinogenicity and reproductive, developmental, acute and chronic toxicity. Data from these testing guidelines usually provide an adequate database upon which to make regulatory decisions. Additional required testing to provide more in-depth characterization of the chemical's neurotoxicity is rare.

Regulatory decisions in the USA and elsewhere may be made on data not generated from an established testing guideline (Tilson et al., 1996). For example, under the US Toxic Substances Control Act, available information (e.g., SAR, results from the literature or other tests) may indicate potential for a compound to produce neurotoxicity.

In this case, the US EPA and the company making the product may negotiate the type of data requirements needed to permit the use of the chemical for industrial purposes.

5.6 Emerging issues

5.6.1 Genetic approaches to neurotoxicology

Techniques to alter or change the germ line have not been used frequently in neurotoxicity risk assessment, although they hold promise for mechanistically based studies (Toews & Morell, 1999). It is thought that genetically altered animals may be differentially sensitive to neurotoxic agents that act via a well delineated mechanism, such as the formation of free radicals, increased intracellular calcium or receptor-mediated effects. The homologous recombination of exogenous DNA with a specific genomic DNA sequence can lead to a recombination that "knocks out" a given gene. Such preparations are frequently performed in mice and have been used in basic studies concerning the role of proteins in the development of the nervous system (Joyner & Guillemont, 1994; Holtmaat et al., 1998). Gene knockouts have been used to study effects mediated through the aryl-hydrocarbon receptor, inflammatory responses, antioxidant metabolism, and binding and metabolism of toxicants such as methylmercury (Toews & Morell, 1999). Transgenic mice with putative targets for neurotoxic agents selectively deleted can be used to test hypotheses about molecular mechanisms (Zhu et al., 1998). The addition of exogenous DNA to the germ line has also been used in toxicology to detect toxicity (Goldsworthy et al., 1994). Genetically altered cell lines may also prove useful in neurotoxicity risk assessment. For example, Durham et al. (1993) produced a cell line by fusing motor neuron-enriched mouse embryonic spinal cord cells with mouse N18TG2 neuroblastoma cells for use in neurotoxicity testing. At the present time, results from studies using genetic approaches to neurotoxicity testing must be interpreted cautiously. Such approaches may provide valuable confirmatory information concerning a chemical's potential mechanism or mode of action, but their application to human neurotoxicity risk assessment is unclear.

5.6.2   Neuroimmunotoxicology

With the discovery that glial cells produce and release factors similar to those released by macrophages in the periphery, a new approach to examining the role of astrocytes and microglia in brain injury has been developed. It is now recognized that immune cytokines play important roles in mediating CNS injury. Although most cells do not constitutively release cytokines within the CNS, inflammation or injury activates neuroglial cells to upregulate the production and secretion of various cytokines during effector phases of immunity (Ari et al., 1990; Benveniste, 1992). Host defence responses are elicited from the organism by any challenge that insults homeostasis, including invasion of pathogens, tissue injury, inflammation, stress, exercise or psychological factors. These responses include changes in the status of the neuroendocrine, cardiovascular, gastric, peripheral nervous and immune systems, behaviour, metabolism and thermoregulation. Many of the effects of cytokines in the brain occur in pathological states when glial cells become activated to proliferate, migrate or express new functional markers (Selmaj et al., 1990; Bourdiol et al., 1991; Lipton, 1992; Giulian, 1993; Giulian & Vaca, 1993). Several inflammatory cytokines are elevated after brain trauma, infectious diseases and neurodegeneration (Hauser et al., 1990; Frei et al., 1993; Sheng et al., 1995). Once induced, cytokines released within the CNS contribute to the injury by influencing vascular permeability (Goldmuntz et al., 1986), inflammatory cell extravasation (Benveniste, 1992) and antigen presentation. Enhanced expression of pro-inflammatory cytokines initiates a complex regulatory cytokine network in the CNS similar to patterns seen in non-neural tissue. In the early stages of an injury response, tumour necrosis factor-alpha, interleukins 1 and 6, and transforming growth factor-beta mediate broad ranges of host responses and affect multiple cell types (Ari et al., 1990; Warren, 1990; Ott et al., 1995; Mattsson et al., 1997). Cytokines can induce or modulate a broad spectrum of cellular responses, including cell adhesion, migration, proliferation, survival, differentiation, replication, secretory function and cell death. Cytokine response in chemical injury has been demonstrated with early stages of demyelination (Mehta et al., 1998) and hippocampal damage (Bruccoleri et al., 1998).

5.6.3   *Endocrine dysfunction/disruption*

There is increased concern that some chemicals in the environment may adversely affect animals and humans by interfering with the production, release, transport, metabolism, binding, action or elimination of natural hormones in the body responsible for developmental processes (Colborn et al., 1994; US EPA, 1998b; EC, 1999; US NRC, 1999). There appear to be a number of chemical-related effects in animals that would be indicative of neuroendocrine disruption, including alterations in reproductive behaviours, body metabolism, sexual differentiation and behavioural development (Tilson, 1998b). Chemicals having possible endocrine-disrupting properties include PCBs, dioxins, chlorinated pesticides, some metals, synthetic steroids, phytoestrogens and triazine herbicides (IUPAC, 1998; US NRC, 1999). Although there is some agreement that environmental chemicals may affect developmental processes in animals, there are uncertainties about associations between exposures to endocrine disruptors and adverse human health effects. For example, environmental exposure to such chemicals occurs in the form of mixtures, which makes it difficult to attribute a specific effect to a particular chemical. In addition, there are concerns about extrapolating results from the laboratory to the field or general environment or results obtained in animal studies to humans. It is also likely that the dose–response curve for alterations in neuroendocrine function is not linear and that some chemicals could have more than one effect occurring at different points on the dose–response curve. Finally, there is a general lack of information concerning the mechanism of action of chemicals that might affect neuroendocrine development. At the present time, the threat to human health following exposure to endocrine disruptors is not known. WHO/IPCS is currently evaluating the scientific literature and preparing a global assessment of the state-of-the-science of endocrine-disrupting chemicals. Research on the possible effects of chemicals on developing neuroendocrine systems and the nervous system should have a high priority.

5.7   Summary

Significant progress has been made in the last 10 years in the area of animal neurotoxicology testing. Batteries of functional tests have been developed, validated and used extensively in neurotoxicological studies. Routine neuropathological procedures are frequently used in concert with functional tests for the initial phases of risk assessment (US EPA, 1991c). Modern neuropathological methods can yield additional and specific information. Many different types of behavioural tests have been used to assess chemical-induced changes in sensory, motor and cognitive function, whereas neurophysiological measures have been standardized to assess chemical-induced sensory and motor function. Recent concern about endocrine-disrupting chemicals has led to the need to consider the neuroendocrine system as a potential site of action in animal studies. Animal models have also been used extensively to study the differential sensitivity of developing organisms to chemical insult. Current guidelines for developmental neurotoxicity testing are complex, and the results are subject to varying interpretations for risk assessment purposes. Although significant advances have been made in the development of *in vitro* procedures to determine the neurotoxicity of chemicals, the use of such tests is generally restricted to cases in which the mechanism or site of action of a chemical is known or predicted.

6. NEUROTOXICITY RISK ASSESSMENT

6.1 Introduction

Risk assessment is an empirically based process used to estimate the risk that exposure of an individual or population to a chemical, physical or biological agent will be associated with an adverse effect. A list of assessments produced by various national and international agencies on specific chemicals is included in ECETOC/UNEP (1996). Risk may be defined as the probability of adverse effects caused under specified conditions by a chemical, physical or biological agent in an organism, a population or an ecological system (OECD/IPCS, 2001). The risk assessment process usually involves four steps: hazard identification, dose–response assessment, exposure assessment and risk characterization (US NRC, 1983; IPCS, 1999). Risk management is the process that applies information obtained through the risk assessment process to determine whether the assessed risk should be reduced and, if so, to what extent. In some cases, risk is the only factor considered in a decision to regulate exposure to a substance. Alternatively, the risk posed by a substance is weighed against social, ethical and medical benefits and economic and technological factors in formulating a risk management decision. The risk-balancing approach is used by some agencies to consider the benefits as well as the risks associated with unrestricted or partially restricted use of a substance.

The purpose of this chapter is to describe the risk assessment process as it has currently evolved in neurotoxicology and present available options for quantitative risk assessment. Assumptions specific to risk assessment for neurotoxicity have been described in section 2.5.

6.2 Hazard identification

Hazard identification is the first stage in hazard assessment or risk assessment, which consists of determining substances of concern and the adverse effects they may inherently have on target systems under certain conditions of exposure, taking into account toxicity data (OECD/IPCS, 2001).

The purpose of hazard identification is to evaluate the weight of evidence for adverse effects in humans based on assessment of all available data, ranging from observations in humans and animal data to an analysis of mechanisms of action and SARs. Each source of information has its advantages and limitations in contributing to the weight-of-evidence approach, but collectively they permit a scientific judgement as to whether the chemical can cause adverse effects.

6.2.1 Human studies

Information obtained through the evaluation of human data often can provide direct identification of neurotoxic hazards. Well documented observational, clinical and epidemiological studies have the clear advantage over studies in animals in providing the most relevant information on human health effects (ECETOC, 1992; US EPA, 1998a). With the exclusion of therapeutic agents, information on effects in humans consists primarily of case reports of accidental exposures, occupational exposures, epidemiological studies and ethically conducted human volunteer studies (see chapter 4).

6.2.2 Animal studies

Because there is generally a lack of adequate human exposure and toxicity data for most chemicals, animal toxicity studies play an important role in hazard identification for risk assessment.

Animal models for many end-points of neurotoxicity are available and widely used for hazard identification. Data from animal studies are commonly extrapolated to humans. For example, if exposure to an agent produces neuropathology in an animal model, damage to a comparable structure in humans is predicted. Similarly, biochemical and physiological effects observed in animals are extrapolated to humans. Agents that produce alterations in the levels of specific enzymes in one animal species generally have the same effect in other species, including humans. Neurophysiological end-points also tend to be affected by the same manipulations across species. Thus, an agent interfering with nerve conduction in an animal study is often assumed to have the same effect in humans. Behavioural studies in animals are also applied to human hazard identification, although the correspondence between methods employed in animals and humans is sometimes not as obvious. However, owing to uncertainties in cross-species extrapolation, a negative result in a single animal species is generally regarded as insufficient evidence of a lack of neurotoxic potential in humans. Positive findings cannot be ignored.

6.2.3 Special issues

6.2.3.1 Animal-to-human extrapolation

The use of animal data to identify hazards for humans is not without controversy. Relative sensitivity across species as well as between sexes is a constant concern. Overly conservative risk assessments, based on the assumption that humans are always more sensitive than a tested animal species, can result in poor risk management decisions. Conversely, an assumption of equivalent sensitivity in a case where humans actually are more sensitive to a given agent can result in underregulation, which might have a negative impact on human health. Interspecies comparisons of kinetics and biotransformation pathways are an important component of interspecies extrapolation.

6.2.3.2 Susceptible populations

A related concern is the use of data collected from adult organisms (animal or human) to predict hazards in potentially more sensitive populations, such as the very young and the elderly. In some cases, identification of neurotoxicity hazard does not generally include subjects from either end of the human life span or from other than healthy subjects. Uncertainty factors are used to adjust for more sensitive populations. In addition, single or multigeneration reproductive studies in animals may provide a source of information on neurological disorders, behavioural changes, autonomic dysfunction, neuroanatomical anomalies and other signs of neurotoxicity in the developing animal.

6.2.3.3 Cumulative toxicity

Cumulative toxicity represents the net change in toxicity resulting from the combined exposure to multiple chemical substances relative to the toxicity caused by each substance alone. While the nature of cumulative toxicity is often identical or similar to an effect caused by one or more of the substances individually, cumulative toxicity among chemicals can be manifested in many ways. Exposure to multiple chemical substances may result in an additive effect, antagonism, synergism or no change in toxic effect caused by any one of the substances alone.

Whether the cumulative toxicity resulting from exposures to pesticides and other chemicals that occur individually as residues in multiple sources such as the diet, air or water will be greater than, equal to or less than the toxicity caused by any of the chemicals alone is dependent on many factors. These include exposure patterns, which result in toxicokinetics/toxicodynamics of each substance causing the common toxic effect, the duration of the common toxic effects and the interactions that take place between substances. For purposes of risk assessment, the cumulative toxicity of multiple chemicals sharing a common mechanism of toxicity (e.g., inhibition of AChE), in the absence of evidence to the contrary, is the effect predicted by summing the exposure to the individual chemicals in the mixture (FQPA, 1996).

.2.3.4   Recovery of function

For the most part, the basic principles of hazard identification are the same for neurotoxicity as for any adverse effect on health. One notable exception, however, concerns the issue of reversibility and the special consideration that must be given to the inherent redundancy and plasticity of the nervous system. Incorporation of a post-dose recovery group into study designs can be of great value to determine the potential for recovery of function.

For many health effects, temporary, as opposed to permanent, morphological changes or other effects are repaired during a true recovery. Damage to many organ systems, if not severe, can be sponta-neously repaired. For example, damaged liver cells that may result in impaired liver function often can be replaced with new cells that function normally. The resulting restoration of liver function can be viewed as recovery. In the CNS, cells generally do not recover from severe damage, and new cells do not replace them. When nervous system recovery is observed, it may represent compensation, requiring activation of cells that were previously performing some other function, reactive synaptogenesis or recovery of moderately injured cells. While a damaged liver may recover as a result of the addition of new cells, severe damage to nervous system cells results in a net loss of neurons. This loss of compensatory capacity may not be noticed for many years, and, when it does appear, it may be manifested in a way seemingly unrelated to the original neurotoxic event. Lack of ability to recover from a neurotoxic event later in life or premature onset of signs of normal aging may result. It is therefore important to consider the possibility that significant damage to the nervous system may persist in experiments where functional effects are not seen. It is particularly likely that relatively slowly evolving damage can allow parallel development of compensating reactions to maintain function.

6.2.4 Characterization of the database and classification schemes

As indicated above, a weight-of-evidence approach to identifying and characterizing neurotoxic hazards entails rigorous evaluation of the quantity, quality and nature of the results of available toxicological and epidemiological studies, information on mechanisms of toxicity and structure–activity analyses. Often, however, individuals charged with hazard assessment are confronted with a collection of imperfect studies providing conflicting data (Barnes & Dourson, 1988).

Several approaches for assessing the weight of evidence are possible, depending on the quality of the database for various toxicological end-points. Two examples are the use of data only from the most sensitive species tested or from species responding most like the human for any given end-point. In assessing the neurotoxicity of therapeutic products, when human data are available and neurotoxic end-points detected in animals can be clinically measured, the human findings supersede those of the non-clinical database.

Assuming that all available evidence is to be included, consider-ations necessary for formulating a conclusion include the relative weights that should be given to positive and negative studies. Risk assessors give positive studies more weight than negative ones, even when the quality of the studies is comparable. Experimental design factors such as the species tested, the number and gender of subjects evaluated, and the duration of the test are given different weights when data from different studies are combined. The route of exposure in a given study and its relevance to expected routes of human exposure are often a weighted factor. The oral route of administration is in general the relevant route for risk assessment of food additives; for workers' protection, however, the main route of exposure is either dermal or inhalation. There may be animal studies that are sufficiently detailed to provide a reliable estimate of the dose–response relationship after oral administration, but few or no data to evaluate the response following dermal or inhalation administration. Extrapolation of data obtained from oral studies to a calculation of a safe inhalation concentration is difficult, and the assessor has to make the judgement that the extrapolation is reliable, e.g., by referring to the internal dose.

The issue of statistical significance is frequently debated. Some argue that an effect occurring at a statistically non-significant level in a study with inadequate statistical power may nevertheless represent a biologically or toxicologically significant event. In general, statistically significant measures that are biologically plausible carry a greater weight in risk assessment. In cases where positive and negative results have been reported in several studies, a meta-analysis may be employed to investigate overall trends.

Several frameworks for assessing the potential of a chemical to produce neurotoxicity have been developed (Johnsen et al., 1992; Hertel, 1996; EC, 1997; US EPA, 1998a; OECD, 1999), and several classification schemes for determining neurotoxic effects have been utilized. In the EU (EC, 1997), substances are not classified as specific neurotoxicants, but are labelled as very toxic, toxic or harmful, based on specific criteria. The criteria are data either from animal studies showing clear signs of CNS depression or from actual observations in humans. Another approach (US EPA, 1998a) focuses on characterizing the sufficiency of available evidence for neurotoxic effects and is not intended to label compounds or generate lists. The purpose of this approach is to provide the risk assessor with the tools to decide whether the available data are sufficient to judge whether or not a human neurotoxic hazard could exist.

In the early 1980s, Spencer & Schaumburg (1985) proposed criteria for the categorization of solvents as human neurotoxicants. They considered a solvent a neurotoxicant in humans if at least three of the following questions are affirmed: (1) Does the substance or mixture produce a consistent pattern of neurological dysfunction in humans? (2) Can this dysfunction be induced in animals under comparable exposure conditions? (3) Are there reproducible lesions in the nervous system or special sense organs of exposed humans or animals? (4) Do the abnormalities satisfactorily account for the neurobehavioural dysfunction?

Johnsen et al. (1992) considered neurotoxicity as a continuum of effects depending on the nature of the chemical, the dose and the duration of exposure. This continuum of signs of neurotoxicity is rank-ordered according to the severity of the observed effects in levels from 1 to 6. The observed effects can encompass morphological, neurological, physiological, electrophysiological and biochemical changes, along with changes in behaviour, symptomatology and neuropsychological status. A range of different measures, tests and techniques exists with which to assess each of these categories of effects. Chemicals are considered more severely neurotoxic if the induced change associated with its exposure is a lasting effect. It should be kept in mind, however, that biochemical changes should not necessarily be interpreted as evidence for neurotoxicity, except in those cases where a chemical is proven neurotoxic with a known mechanism of action (e.g., organophosphate-induced peripheral neuropathy). Finally, the existence of irreversible subjective symptoms alone in humans should be supported by experimental data.

The approach by Johnsen et al. (1992) is similar in concept to the one used by IARC (1987) for the classification of carcinogens. It first evaluates the quality and credibility of the existing animal and human studies on a chemical and then proceeds to classify the neurotoxicity of the chemical. There are four different levels of evidence: *Sufficient Evidence* (well conducted, high-quality studies describing severe effects), *Limited Evidence* (well conducted studies demonstrating low to moderate effects or less well conducted studies showing severe effects), *Inadequate Evidence* (poorly conducted studies having marginal relevance to neurotoxicology or studies reporting low to moderate effects) and *Negative Evidence* (well conducted studies showing no neurotoxic effects). After an examination of the nature of the neurotoxicity, the chemical is then classified into one of the following five categories: *Neurotoxic to Humans* (sufficient evidence from human studies or limited evidence from humans supported by sufficient evidence from animal experiments), *Probably Neurotoxic to Humans* (limited evidence from human and animal studies or sufficient evidence from animal studies and inadequate evidence from human studies or supporting evidence from *in vitro* tests or SAR analyses), *Possibly Neurotoxic to Humans* (human data are negative and animal data are sufficient to negative), *Probably Not Neurotoxic to Humans* (based on negative data in humans and negative or inadequate evidence from animal studies) or *Cannot Be Classified* (probably not neurotoxic in humans based on negative evidence in humans and negative or inadequate evidence from animal studies). The neurotoxic potency of a chemical is based on a description of the dose–effect relationship. When a functional dose–response relationship is established, it is generally possible to estimate a no-effect level or a lowest-observed-effect level, which can be used as a measurement of toxic potential and to set exposure limits. Simonsen et al. (1995) reported on the use of this classification approach to evaluate the neurotoxic potential for 79 compounds. These authors found that 27 of the selected chemicals would be classified as neurotoxic according to this approach, while 24 were classified as probable human neurotoxicants, and 14 were considered possible neurotoxicants.

In another approach, Ladefoged et al. (1995) classified chemicals on the basis of inherent neurotoxicological properties into the following categories: *Category 1* — Compounds known to cause serious damage to the nervous system (sufficient evidence to establish a causal relationship between human exposure and impaired nervous system function); *Category 2* — Substances that should be regarded as if they cause serious damage to the nervous system (sufficient evidence to support a strong association between human exposure to the substance and impaired nervous system function based on (a) clear evidence in animal studies of impaired nervous system function occurring at around the same dose levels as other toxicity, which is not a secondary non-specific consequence of the other toxic effects, and (b) other relevant information, such as *in vitro* test results and quantitative SAR analysis); and *Category 3* — Substances that cause concern for the human nervous system (generally based on (a) results in appropriate animal studies that suggest the possibility of impaired nervous system function in the absence of other toxic effects or (b) evidence of impaired function occurring at around the same dose levels as other toxic effects, but not a secondary non-specific consequence of the other toxic effects).

Recently, Spencer et al. (2000) proposed the following updated set of criteria for the positive identification of neurotoxic chemicals: (1) presence of the suspected agent is confirmed by history and either environmental or clinical chemical analysis; (2) severity and temporal onset of the condition are commensurate with duration and level of exposure: (3) the condition is self-limiting, and clinical improvement follows removal from exposure; (4) clinical features display a consistent pattern that corresponds to previous cases; and (5) development of a satisfactory corresponding experimental *in vivo* or *in vitro* model is absolute proof of causation. In conjunction with these criteria, a rating system is used to assess the strength of association between exposure to an agent and the neurotoxic effect.

The US EPA approach is to define two broad categories, sufficient evidence and insufficient evidence of a human health neurotoxic hazard (US EPA, 1998a). The sufficient evidence category includes data that collectively provide enough information to judge whether or not a human neurotoxic hazard could exist. This category may include both human and experimental animal evidence. Sufficient human evidence is based on positive neurotoxic effects in epidemiological studies, e.g., case–control and cohort studies. A well documented case report in conjunction with other supporting evidence may also be judged as sufficient evidence. Sufficient evidence of potential neurotoxic risk may also come from experimental animal studies. Limited human data may be used to support positive effects in animal studies. The minimum evidence necessary to judge that a potential hazard exists would be data demonstrating an adverse, neurotoxic effect in a single appropriate, well executed study in a single experimental animal species. The minimum evidence needed to judge that a potential hazard does not exist would include data from an appropriate number of end-points from more than one study and two species showing no adverse neurotoxic effects at doses that were minimally toxic in terms of producing an adverse effect of some type. Information on pharmacokinetics, mechanisms or known properties of the chemical class may also be used to strengthen the evidence.

The second category, i.e., insufficient evidence, includes data from which there is less than the minimum evidence for identifying whether or not a neurotoxic hazard exists, such as agents for which there are no data on neurotoxicity or agents with databases from studies in animals or humans that are limited by study design or conduct (e.g., inadequate conduct, too few samples, lack of quantification of symptoms). Many general toxicity studies are considered insufficient because of the conduct of clinical observations or the number of samples taken for histopathology of the nervous system. A battery of negative toxicity studies with these shortcomings would be regarded as providing insufficient evidence of the lack of a neurotoxic effect of the chemical. Most screening studies based on simple observations in isolation provide insufficient evaluation of many functions and are also considered insufficient evidence. Information on SAR or data from *in vitro* studies in isolation would also fall into this category. Although such information would be insufficient by itself to proceed further in the assessment, it could be used to support requirements for additional testing.

This approach recognizes that chemicals may have effects on both the structure and function of the nervous system (Tilson et al., 1995). Chemical-induced changes in morphology (neuropathology) are considered to be neurotoxic. Functional changes include alterations in behaviour, neurophysiology and neurochemistry. Irreversible functional changes are viewed as adverse effects. Reversible functional changes could be adverse under certain experimental circumstances (Tilson et al., 1995). For example, some chemicals may interfere with motor function, which could affect performance in the workplace. If it could be demonstrated that such an effect occurred at occupationally or environmentally relevant doses or concentrations, then the reversible functional change could be considered adverse. In other cases, reversible functional changes are associated with a known mechanism of action. For example, cholinesterase-inhibiting pesticides inhibit AChE, which leads to a syndrome associated with cholinergic over-stimulation. Although the clinical signs associated with inhibition of cholinesterase enzyme are short-lived, they can be deadly and must be considered adverse.

In other cases, reversible functional changes may co-vary with a known neurotoxic effect. For example, chemical-induced injury to the nervous system can produce an astrocyte response and increase the expression of cellular proteins such as GFAP. Although the increase in GFAP may be transient, such changes would be viewed with concern because they are associated with a known adverse effect. Effects that appear to be reversible should always be evaluated cautiously and in light of all other data available. While the nervous system has a limited capacity for regeneration, it does have the capacity to adjust and compensate for damage by the surviving cells, assuming additional functions. Thus, the inability to detect an effect at a later testing time may be indicative not of a system returned to normal but rather of a system that has compensated for earlier damage. Under these conditions, the question remains as to whether the system has reserve capacity that would allow for it to compensate for a secondary damage or if instead such capacity is no longer available and the system is now more vulnerable to later injury. Given the relatively crude sensitivity of the screening test systems now routinely used, additional test methods and further investigation may be required to "unmask" any underlying damage.

These examples of classification schemes have been helpful in standardizing and communicating the assessments of hazard identification for neurotoxic end-points. However, each scheme has strengths and weaknesses. In addition to the classifications themselves, narrative statements describing the nature and confidence in the evidence based on strengths and limitations of the database are important. Correlated measures of neurotoxicity (e.g., between functional and morphological effects) can strengthen the evidence for a potential human health hazard. Such correlations can also support a coherent and logical link between effects and cellular mechanisms.

6.3   Dose–response assessment

Dose–response assessment consists of analysing the relationship between the total amount of a chemical, physical or biological agent administered to, taken by or absorbed by an organism and the changes developed in it in reaction to the agent and inferences derived from such an analysis with respect to larger groups of organisms or the entire population (OECD/IPCS, 2001). Approaches to quantification of dose–response effects vary according to the scope and purpose of the assessments (IPCS, 1987, 1994).

Dose–response assessment is a critical part of the qualitative characterization of a chemical's potential to produce neurotoxicity and involves the description of the dose–response relationship in the available data (IPCS, 1999). Human studies covering a range of exposures are rarely available; therefore, animal data are typically used for estimating exposure levels likely to produce adverse effects in humans. Evidence for a dose–response relationship is an important criterion in establishing a neurotoxic effect, although this analysis may be limited when based on standard studies using three dose groups or fewer. The evaluation of dose–response relationships includes identifying effective dose levels as well as doses associated with no increase in incidence of adverse effects when compared with controls. Much of the focus is on identifying the critical effect(s) observed at the lowest-observed-adverse-effect level (LOAEL) and the no-observed-adverse-effect-level (NOAEL) associated with that effect. The NOAEL is defined as the highest dose at which there is no statistically or biologically significant increase in the frequency of an adverse neurotoxic effect when compared with the appropriate control group in a database characterized as having sufficient evidence for use in a risk assessment. The LOAEL is defined as the lowest dose at which there is a statistically or biologically significant adverse effect.

The dose–response assessment defines the range of doses that are neurotoxic for a given agent, species, route of exposure and duration of exposure. In addition to these considerations, pharmacokinetic factors and other aspects that might influence comparisons with human exposure scenarios should be taken into account. For example, dose–response curves may exhibit not only monotonic but also U-shaped or inverted U-shaped functions (Davis & Svendsgaard, 1989). Such curves are hypothesized to reflect multiple mechanisms of action, the presence of homeostatic mechanisms or activation of compensatory or protective mechanisms. In addition to considering the shape of the dose–response curve, it should also be recognized that neurotoxic effects vary in terms of nature and severity across dose or exposure level. At high levels of exposure, frank lesions accompanied by severe functional impairment may be observed. Such effects are widely accepted as adverse. At progressively lower levels of exposure, however, the lesions may become less severe and the impairments less obvious. At levels of exposure near the NOAEL and LOAEL, the effects will often be mild, possibly reversible and inconsistently found.

In addition, the end-points showing responses may be at levels of organization below the whole organism (e.g., neurochemical or electrophysiological end-points). The adversity of such effects can be disputed (e.g., plasma cholinesterase inhibition), yet it is such effects that are likely to be the focus of risk assessment decisions. To the extent possible, this document provides guidance on determining the adversity of neurotoxic effects. However, the identification of a critical adverse effect often requires considerable professional judgement and should consider factors such as the biological plausibility of the effect, the evidence of a dose–effect continuum and the likelihood for progression of the effect with continued exposure.

The use of mechanistic data in characterizing risk is of current concern to risk assessors. Becking (1995) suggested that mechanistic data could be used as an alternative to the traditional threshold, NOAEL methodology used in risk assessment. Lotti (1995) demonstrated, using an organophosphate-induced polyneuropathy model, three main areas of extrapolation where mechanistic data could be incorporated into the current risk assessment process and reduce uncertainty, including extrapolation from (1) animals to humans, (2) high to low dose levels and (3) disintegrated systems to complex systems.

Predictions of risk are frequently based on incomplete data, and risk assessment processes are generally conservative, i.e., designed to protect human health. Hazard characterization leads to the identification of a neurotoxic effect occurring at some exposure level. Quantitative risk assessment attempts to determine if the effect in question would occur at an exposure level that would endanger human health. This process typically involves selecting an exposure level that is less than that known to produce an adverse health effect, i.e., NOAEL, and dividing the level by some factor or factors to arrive at what is considered to be a "safe" or "acceptable" level of exposure. Lehman & Fitzhugh (1954) described the first safety factor approach as it relates to the regulation of food additives for human consumption. A safety factor is a number that is applied to an observed or estimated concentration or dose to arrive at a criterion or standard that is considered safe (OECD/IPCS, 2001). Lehman & Fitzhugh (1954) recommended a safety factor of 100, which appeared to be high enough to reduce the hazard of food additives to a minimum and also permit the use of the chemicals commercially. The uncertainty factor was based on uncertainties of extrapolating from animals to humans and variation in human responsiveness to chemical exposure. The NOAEL divided by the safety factor was termed the acceptable daily intake or ADI. The ADI may be defined as the maximum amount of a substance to which someone may be exposed daily over the life span without appreciable risk (OECD/IPCS, 2001). The term tolerable daily intake (TDI) has also been used. According to the US Consumer Product Safety Commission (Babich, 1998), an exposure to a chemical during "reasonably forseeable handling and use" that exceeds the ADI is considered hazardous.

Subsequent to the general use of the ADI approach, some risk assessors began to develop the concept of reference doses (RfDs) or reference concentrations (RfCs) for inhalation exposures (Doull, 1990). RfDs or RfCs are estimates of doses or concentrations that would be safe if consumed over a lifetime. In this approach, several uncertainty factors are utilized, and the magnitude is set at a default value of 10, which could be reduced to as low as 1 depending on the quality of the available data. Uncertainty factors are numbers applied to an observed or estimated toxic concentration or dose to accommodate the fact that the present knowledge of certain parameters may be insufficient to ensure absolute precision in the risk assessment (OECD/IPCS, 2001). Like the ADI approach, uncertainty factors are included for variations in sensitivity within the human population and the possibility that humans may be up to 10 times more sensitive than laboratory animals (total factor of 100). Additional uncertainty factors of 10 are used for less-than-lifetime exposures of the animal and in cases where a LOAEL is used in the absence of a NOAEL. Finally, a factor of 10 may also be used if there are deficiencies in the database. The dose–response for an average human (population mean) occurs at doses 10-fold lower than those in animals. Probabilistic approaches can be used to define the likelihood that the 10-fold factor may be an over- or underestimation (Slob & Pieters, 1998). It is considered that the 100-fold factor is composed of two factors of 10; each factor of 10 has to allow for differences in toxicokinetics and toxicodynamics (IPCS, 1994; Renwick & Lazarus, 1998). The size of the final uncertainty factor used will vary from agent to agent and will require the exercise of scientific judgement, taking into account interspecies differences, the shape of the dose–response curve and the neurotoxicity end-points observed. Barnes & Dourson (1988) provided a more complete description of the calculation, use and significance of RfDs in setting exposure limits for toxic agents by the oral route. Jarabek et al. (1990) provided a more complete description of the calculation, use and significance of RfCs in setting exposure limits for toxic agents in air. Neurotoxicity can result from acute, shorter-term exposures, and it may be appropriate in some cases, e.g., for air pollutants or water contaminants, to set shorter-term exposure limits for neurotoxicity as well as for other non-cancer health effects.

The ADI/RfD/RfC approaches rely on the determination of a NOAEL or LOAEL. However, several limitations in the use of the NOAEL have been identified and described (e.g., Crump, 1984; Barnes & Dourson, 1988). For example, the NOAEL is derived from a single end-point from a single study (the critical study) and ignores both the slope of the dose–response function and baseline variability in the end-point of concern. Because the baseline variability is not taken into account, the NOAEL from a study using small group sizes may be higher than the NOAEL from a similar study in the same species that uses larger group sizes. The NOAEL is also directly dependent on the dose spacing used in the study. Finally, and perhaps most importantly, use of the NOAEL does not allow estimates or extrapolation of risk to lower dose levels. Because of these and other limitations in the NOAEL approach, it has been proposed that mathematical curve-fitting techniques (Crump, 1984; Gaylor & Slikker, 1990; Glowa, 1991; Glowa & MacPhail, 1995; US EPA, 1995; Slikker et al., 1996) should be compared with the NOAEL procedure in calculating the RfD or RfC. These techniques typically apply a mathematical function that describes the dose–response relationship and then interpolate to a level of exposure associated with a small increase in effect over that occurring in the control group or under baseline conditions. One example is the benchmark dose (BMD), which has been defined as a lower confidence limit on the effective dose associated with some defined level of effect, e.g., a 5% or 10% increase in response in excess of background. Mutti & Smargiassi (1998) compared the results of a BMD approach and the traditional approach based on LOAELs and NOAELs in assessing the effects of exposure to some neurotoxic organic solvents and metals. Between these approaches, variation was seen in the resulting neurotoxic thresholds estimated for each chemical examined. For example, in comparison to the estimated thresholds found from the BMD, the NOAEL-based estimate was about the same for manganese, double for lead and half as high for styrene. Others have also compared the procedures and results of the risk assessments of neurotoxicants (e.g., MPTP) using the BMD and the traditional NOAEL/LOAEL approach (e.g., Slikker et al., 1996). In addition to disagreements about the derivation procedures utilized (e.g., Crofton et al., 1996; Gaylor & Slikker, 1996), differences in the resulting acceptable total dose of exposure (or threshold) between these approaches also emerged. Thus, additional work is needed to compare different risk assessment approaches and to validate the more novel ones.

Many neurotoxic end-points provide continuous measures of response, such as response speed, NCV, IQ score, degree of enzyme inhibition or the accuracy of task performance. Although it is possible to impose a dichotomy on a continuous effects distribution and to classify some level of response as "affected'" and the remainder as "unaffected," it may be very difficult and inappropriate to establish such clear distinctions, because such a dichotomy would misrepresent the true nature of the neurotoxic response. Alternatively, quantitative models designed to analyse continuous effect variables may be preferable. Other techniques that allow this approach, with trans- formation of the information into estimates of the incidence or frequency of affected individuals in a population, have been proposed (Crump, 1984; Gaylor & Slikker, 1990; Glowa & MacPhail, 1995). Categorical regression analysis has been proposed, since it can evaluate different types of data and derive estimates for short-term exposures (Rees & Hattis, 1994). Decisions about the most appropriate approach require professional judgement, taking into account the biological nature of the continuous effect variable and its distribution in the population under study.

Although dose–response functions in neurotoxicology are gen- erally linear or monotonic, curvilinear functions, especially U-shaped or inverted U-shaped curves, have been reported, as noted above. Dose–response analyses should consider the uncertainty that U-shaped dose–response functions might contribute to the estimate of the NOAEL/LOAEL or BMD. Typically, estimates of the NOAEL/ LOAEL are taken from the lowest part of the dose–response curve associated with impaired function or adverse effect.

6.4 Exposure assessment

Exposure assessment describes the magnitude, duration, frequency and routes of exposure to the agent of interest (IPCS, 1999). The OECD/IPCS project on the harmonization of hazard/risk assessment terminology has defined exposure assessment as consisting of a quantitative and qualitative analysis of the amount of a chemical or biological agent, including its derivatives, that may be present in a given environment and the inference of the possible consequences it may have for a given population of particular concern (OECD/IPCS, 2001). This information may come from hypothetical values, models or actual experimental values, including ambient environmental sampling results (Chern et al., 1995).

The exposure assessment should include an exposure characterization that provides a statement of the purpose, scope, level of detail and approach used in the exposure assessment. Estimates of exposure and dose by pathway and route for individuals, population segments and populations in a manner appropriate for the intended risk characterization should also be presented. An evaluation of the overall level of confidence in the estimate of exposure and dose and the conclusions drawn should be made, and the results of the exposure assessment should be communicated to the risk assessor, who can then use the exposure characterization, along with the hazard and dose–response characterizations, to develop an overall assessment of the potential for a chemical to produce a hazard for humans.

A number of considerations are relevant to exposure assessment for neurotoxicants. An appropriate evaluation of exposure should consider the potential for exposure via ingestion, inhalation and dermal penetration from relevant sources of exposures, including multiple avenues of intake from the same source. In addition, neurotoxic effects may result from short-term (acute), high-concentration exposures as well as from longer-term (subchronic), lower-level exposures. Neurotoxic effects may occur after a period of time following initial exposure or be obfuscated by repair mechanisms or apparent tolerance. The type and severity of effect may depend significantly on the pattern of exposure rather than on the average dose over a long period of time. For this reason, exposure assessments for neurotoxicants may be much more complicated than those for long-latency effects such as carcinogenicity. It is rare for sufficient data to be available to construct such patterns of exposure or dose, and professional judgement may be necessary to evaluate exposure to neurotoxic agents.

In the case of developmental neurotoxicity, there are a number of important questions concerning exposure. For example, the possible routes by which the fetus may be exposed could be a significant factor. Exposure of the fetus to a chemical depends on maternal absorption, distribution, metabolism, and placental metabolism and transfer of the parent compound or its metabolites. Furthermore, the fetus may have some capability of metabolizing or excreting the chemical. It is also possible that a chemical could indirectly affect the fetus by directly affecting the mother. In the case of newborns, exposure to chemicals could occur via the breast milk, whereas children display a number of behavioural traits that could increase their exposure by oral ingestion. The exposure assessment should determine the extent to which pregnant women, infants or children would be expected to be exposed to a chemical. This information could prove significant in the risk characterization of a chemical.

6.5 Risk characterization

6.5.1 Introduction

Risk characterization is the qualitative and/or quantitative estimation, including attendant uncertainties, of the severity and probability of occurrence of known and potential adverse effects of a substance in a given population, based on hazard identification, dose–response assessment and exposure assessment (OECD/IPCS, 2001). Risk characterizations typically consist of an integrative analysis and a summary of all findings. The integrative analysis (1) involves integration of all the toxicological results from the hazard characterization and dose–response analysis with the human exposure estimates, (2) provides an evaluation of the overall quality of the assessment and the degree of confidence in the estimates of neurotoxic risk and conclusions drawn, and (3) describes neurotoxic risk in terms of the nature and extent of harm.

6.5.2 Integration

In developing the hazard identification, dose–response analysis and exposure portions of the risk assessment, the assessor must take into account many judgements concerning human relevance of the toxicity data, including the appropriateness of the various animal models for which data are available and the route, timing and duration of exposure relative to expected human exposure. These judgements should be summarized at each stage of the risk assessment process (e.g., the biological relevance of anatomical variations in the hazard characterization process, or the influence of species differences in metabolic patterns in the dose–response analysis). In integrating the information from the assessment, the risk assessor must determine if some of these judgements have implications for other portions of the assessment and whether the various components of the assessment are compatible.

The risk characterization should not only examine the judgements but also explain the constraints of available data and the state of knowledge about the phenomena studied in making them, including (1) the qualitative conclusions about the likelihood that the chemical may pose a specific hazard to human health, the nature of the observed effects, under what conditions (route, dose levels, time and duration) of exposure these effects occur, and whether the health-related data are sufficient to use in a risk assessment; (2) a discussion of the dose–response characteristics of the critical effects(s), data such as the shapes and slopes of the dose–response curves for the various endpoints, the rationale behind the determination of the NOAEL and LOAEL and calculation of the BMD, and the assumptions underlying the estimation of the ADI/RfD/RfC; and (3) the estimates of the magnitude of human exposure; the route, duration and pattern of the exposure; relevant pharmacokinetics; and the number and characteristics of the population(s) exposed.

If data to be used in a risk characterization are from a route of exposure other than the expected human exposure route, then pharmacokinetic data should be used, if available, to make extrapolations across routes of exposure.

The level of confidence in the hazard characterization should be stated to the extent possible, including the appropriate category regarding sufficiency of the health-related data. A comprehensive risk assessment ideally includes information on a variety of end-points that provide insight into the full spectrum of potential neurotoxicological responses. A profile that integrates both human and test species data and incorporates a broad range of potential adverse neurotoxic effects provides more confidence in a risk assessment for a given agent.

The ability to describe the nature of the potential human exposure is important to predict when certain outcomes can be anticipated and the likelihood of permanence or reversibility of the effect. An important part of this effort is a description of the nature of the exposed population and the potential for sensitive, highly susceptible or highly exposed populations. For example, the consequences of exposure of the developing individual compared with those of adult exposure can differ markedly and can influence whether the effects are transient or permanent. Other considerations relative to human exposures might include the likelihood of exposures to other agents, concurrent disease and nutritional status.

3.5.3 *Quality of the database*

The risk characterization should summarize the kinds of data brought together in the analysis and the reasoning on which the assessment is based. The description should convey the major strengths and weaknesses of the assessment that arise from availability of data and the current limits of our understanding of the mechanisms of toxicity.

A health risk assessment is only as good as its component parts, i.e., hazard characterization, dose–response analysis and exposure assessment. Confidence in the results of a risk assessment is, thus, a function of confidence in the results of the analysis of these elements. Each of these elements should have its own characterization as a part of the assessment. Within each characterization, the important uncertainties of the analysis and interpretation of the data should be explained, and the risk manager should be given a clear picture of the consensus or lack of consensus that exists about significant aspects of the assessment. Whenever more than one view is supported by the data and choosing between them is difficult, all views should be presented.

If one has been selected over the others, the rationale should be given; if not, then all should be presented as plausible alternative results. Certainly, individual differences in metabolizing enzymes may be the basis for inter-individual variability. However, inter-individual responses may also be due to pharmacodynamic factors such as differences in brain content of protective enzymes (e.g., glutathione transferase) (Baez et al., 1997).

6.5.4 Descriptors of neurotoxicity risk

There are a number of ways to describe risks. Several ways that are relevant to describing risks for neurotoxicity are listed below.

6.5.4.1 Estimation of the number of individuals

The RfD or RfC is taken to be a chronic exposure level at or below which no significant risk occurs. Therefore, presentation of the population in terms of those at or below the RfD or RfC ("not at risk") and above the RfD or RfC ("may be at risk") may be useful information for risk managers. This method is particularly useful to a risk manager considering possible actions to ameliorate risk for a population. If the number of persons in the at-risk category can be estimated, then the number of persons removed from the at-risk category after a contemplated action is taken can be used as an indication of the efficacy of the action.

6.5.4.2 Presentation of specific scenarios

Presenting specific scenarios in the form of "what if?" questions is particularly useful to give perspective to the risk manager, especially where criteria, tolerance limits or media quality limits are being set. The question being asked in these cases is, at this proposed exposure limit, what would be the resulting risk for neurotoxicity above the RfD or RfC?

6.5.4.3 Risk characterization for highly exposed individuals

This measure describes the magnitude of concern at the upper end of the exposure distribution. This allows risk managers to evaluate whether certain individuals are at disproportionately or unacceptably high risk.

The objective of looking at the upper end of the exposure distribution is to derive a realistic estimate of a relatively highly exposed individual or individuals. This measure could be addressed by identifying a specified upper percentile of exposure in the population or by estimating the exposure of the highest exposed individual(s). Whenever possible, it is important to express the number of individuals who comprise the selected highly exposed group and discuss the potential for exposure at still higher levels.

If population data are absent, it will often be possible to describe a scenario representing high-end exposures using upper-percentile or judgement-based values for exposure variables. In these instances, caution should be used not to compound a substantial number of high-end values for variables if a "reasonable" exposure estimate is to be achieved.

5.4.4 *Risk characterization for highly sensitive or susceptible individuals*

This measure identifies populations sensitive or susceptible to the effect of concern. Sensitive or susceptible individuals are those within the exposed population at increased risk of expressing the toxic effect. All stages of nervous system maturation might be considered highly sensitive or susceptible, but certain subpopulations can sometimes be identified because of critical periods for exposure, e.g., infants and children (IPCS, 1984, 1999). The aged population is considered to be at particular risk because of the limited ability of the nervous system to regenerate or compensate to neurotoxic insult (IPCS, 1994).

In general, not enough is understood about the mechanisms of toxicity to identify sensitive subgroups for all agents, although factors such as nutrition (e.g., vitamin B), personal habits (e.g., smoking, alcohol consumption, illicit drug abuse), or pre-existing disease (e.g., diabetes, neurological diseases, sexually transmitted diseases, polymorphisms for certain metabolic enzymes) may predispose some individuals to be more sensitive to the neurotoxic effects of specific agents. Gender-related differences in response to neurotoxicants have been noted, but these appear to be related to gender-dependent toxico-dynamic or toxicokinetic factors.

Despite the fact that there are limited data available, it is assumed that an uncertainty factor of 10 for intra-population variability, based on differing toxicokinetics and toxicodynamics, will be able to accommodate differences in sensitivity between various subpopulations, including children and the elderly. However, in cases where it can be demonstrated that a factor of 10 does not afford adequate protection, another uncertainty factor may be considered in conducting the risk assessment (FQPA, 1996).

6.5.4.5 Other risk descriptors

In risk characterization, dose–response information and the human exposure estimates may be combined either by comparing the RfD or RfC and the human exposure estimate or by calculating the margin of exposure (MOE). The MOE is the ratio of the NOAEL from the most appropriate or sensitive species to the estimated human exposure level. If a NOAEL is not available, a LOAEL may be used in calculating the MOE. Alternatively, a BMD may be compared with the estimated human exposure level to obtain the MOE. Considerations for the evaluation of the MOE are similar to those for the uncertainty factor applied to the LOAEL/NOAEL or the BMD. The MOE is presented along with a discussion of the adequacy of the database, including the nature and quality of the hazard and exposure data, the number of species affected and the dose–response information.

The RfD or RfC comparison with the human exposure estimate and the calculation of the MOE are conceptually similar but are used in different regulatory situations. The choice of approach depends on several factors, including the statute involved, the situation being addressed, the database used and the needs of the decision maker. The RfD or RfC and the MOE are considered along with other risk assessment and risk management issues in making risk management decisions, but the scientific issues that must be taken into account in establishing them have been addressed here.

If the MOE is equal to or more than the uncertainty factor multiplied by any modifying factor used as a basis for an RfD or RfC, then the need for regulatory concern is likely to be small. Although these methods of describing risk do not actually estimate risks *per se,* they give the risk manager some sense of how close the exposures are to levels of concern.

6.6 Summary

Risk assessment processes for new and existing chemicals have been published and put into use by several different countries in Europe, the Americas and Asia for several years. These processes are relatively similar and include consideration of hazard identification, dose–response evaluation, exposure assessment and risk characterization. Guidance on principles to be used for risk assessment for neurotoxicity has been published by OECD, the US EPA and the EC. The approaches discussed in these documents differ, in that one approach focuses on characterizing the sufficiency of available evidence for determining if a neurotoxic effect exists, while the other focuses on defining a process for assigning chemicals to groups depending on available evidence. In comparing the general risk assessment guidance documents and the specific neurotoxicity guidance documents as well as other information available from the fields of neurobiology and neurotoxicology, the application of risk assessment principles for neurotoxicants is similar to that of other non-cancer end-points, except that issues of reversibility, compensation and recovery of function in the nervous system require special consideration. This document provides guidance on neurotoxicity risk assessment at a broad international level. As for other fields of risk assessment, a key to providing sound neurotoxicity assessments is the quality of the underlying database.

REFERENCES

Aasly J, Storsaeter O, Nilsen G, Smevik O, & Rinck P (1993) Minor structural brain changes in young drug abusers: A magnetic resonance study. Acta Neurol Scand, 87(3): 210–214.

Abou-Donia MB (1995) Organophosphorous pesticides. In: Chang LW & Dyer RS ed. Handbook of neurotoxicology. New York, Marcel Dekker, pp 419–474.

Adams J & Buelke-Sam J (1981) Behavioral testing of the postnatal animal: Testing and methods development. In: Kimmel CA & Buelke-Sam J ed. Developmental toxicology. New York, Raven Press, pp 233–238.

Agnew J & Masten VL (1994) Neuropsychological assessment of occupational neurotoxic exposure. In: Bleeker ML & Hansen JA ed. Occupational neurology and clinical neurotoxicology. Baltimore, Maryland, Williams and Wilkins, pp 113–132.

Aibara K (1986) Introduction to the diagnosis of mycotoxicosis. In: Richards JL & Thurston JR ed. Diagnosis of mycotoxicoses. Dordrecht, Martinus Nijhoff Publishers, pp 3–8.

Alder S & Zbinden G (1983) Neurobehavioural tests in single- and repeated-dose toxicity studies in small rodents. Arch Toxicol, 54(1): 1–23.

Ali SF & Slikker W (1995) Basic biochemical approaches in neurotoxicology: Assessment of neurotransmitters and neuroreceptors. In: Chang LW & Slikker W ed. Neurotoxicology: Approaches and methods. New York, Academic Press, pp 385–398.

Altenkirch H (1982) Schnuffelsucht und Schnuffelneuropathie. In: Bauer H, Baumgartner G, Davison AN, & Ganshirt H ed. Schriftenreihe Neurologie. Berlin-Heidelberg, Springer-Verlag, vol 23.

Altenkirch H, Stoltenburg-Didinger S, & Koeppel C (1988) The neurotoxicological aspects of the toxic oil syndrome (TOS) in Spain. Toxicology, 49: 25–34.

Altmann L, Schardt H, & Wiegand H (1991) Selective effects of acute repeated solvent exposure on the visual system. Arbete Hälsa (Work Health), 35: 67–69.

Altmann L, Sveinsson K, Krämer U, Winneke G, & Wiegand H (1997) Assessment of neurophysiologic and neurobehavioral effects of environmental pollutants in 5- and 6-year-old children. Environ Res, 73(1–2): 125–131.

Amaducci L, Formo KL, & Eng LF (1981) Glial fibrillary acidic protein in cryogenic lesions of the rat brain. Neurosci Lett, 21: 27–32.

Amler RW, Anger WK, & Sizemore OJ (1995) Adult environmental neurobehavioral test battery. Training manual. Atlanta, Georgia, Agency for Toxic Substances and Disease Registry, pp 1–360.

Anand-Kumar TC, David GF, Sankaranarayanan A, Puri V, & Sundram KR (1982) Pharmacokinetics of progesterone after its administration to ovariectomized rhesus monkeys by injection, infusion, or nasal spraying. Proc Natl Acad Sci, 79: 4185–4189.

Andersen ME, Clewell HJ, Gargas ML, MacNaughton MG, Reitz RH, Nolan RJ, & McKenna MJ (1991) Physiologically based pharmacokinetic modeling with dichloromethane, its metabolite, carbon monoxide, and blood carboxyhemoglobin in rats and humans. Toxicol Appl Pharmacol, 108: 14–27.

Anger WK (1984) Neurobehavioural testing of chemicals; impact on recommended standard. Neurobehav Toxicol Teratol, **6**: 147–153.

Anger WK (1990) Human neurobehavioural toxicology testing. In: Russell RW, Flattau PE, & Pope AM ed. Behavioural measures of neurotoxicity. Washington, DC, National Academy Press.

Anger WK, Cassito MG, Liang Y-X, Amador R, Hooisma J, Chrislip DW, Mergler D, Keifer M, & Hortnagl J (1993) Comparison of performance from three continents on the WHO-recommended Neurobehavioral Core Test Battery (NCTB). Environ Res, **62**: 125–147.

Anger WK, Letz R, Chrislip D, Frumkin H, Hudnell K, Russo JM, Chappell W, & Hutchinson L (1994) Neurobehavioral test methods for environmental health studies of adults. Neurotoxicol Teratol, **16**: 489–497.

Anger WK, Sizemore OJ, Grossman SJ, Glasser JA, Letz R, & Bowler R (1997) Human neurobehavioral research methods: Impact of subject variables. Environ Res, **73**: 18–41.

Anger W, Liang Y-X, Nell V, Seong-Kyu K, Cole D, Bazyleqicz-Walczak B, Rohlman DS, Sizemore OJ (2000) Lessons learned — 15 years of the WHO-NCTB: A review. Neurotoxicology, **21**: 837–846.

Annau Z & Eccles CU (1986) Prenatal exposure. In: Annau A ed. Neurobehavioural toxicology. Baltimore, Maryland, Johns Hopkins University Press, pp 153–169.

Anon (1986) Leads from the MMWR. Aldicarb food poisoning from contaminated melons — California. J Am Med Assoc, **256**: 175–176.

Araki S & Murata K (1993) Determination of evoked potentials in occupational and environmental medicine: A review. Environ Res, **63**: 133–147.

Araki S, Yokoyama K, & Murata K (1997) Neurophysiological methods in occupational and environmental health: Methodology and recent findings. Environ Res, **73**: 42–51.

Arenander AT & deVellis J (1983) Frontiers of glial physiology. In: Rosenberg R ed. The clinical neurosciences. New York, Churchill Livingstone, pp 53–91.

Arezzo JC, Schaumburg HH, & Petersen CA (1983) Rapid screening for peripheral neuropathy: A field study with the Optacon. Neurology, **33**(5): 626–629.

Ari K, Lee F, Miyajima A, Shoichiro M, Arai N, & Yokota T (1990) Cytokines: Coordinators of immune and inflammatory responses. Annu Rev Biochem, **59**: 783–836.

Arlien-Søborg P (1992) Solvent neurotoxicity. Boca Raton, Florida, CRC Press.

Armstrong BK, White E, & Saracci R (1992) Principles of exposure measurement in epidemiology. New York, Oxford University Press.

Arrighi HM & Hertz-Picciotto I (1994) The evolving concept of the healthy worker effect. Epidemiology, **5**: 189–196.

Arvidson B (1994) A review of axonal transport of metals. Toxicology, **11**: 1–14.

Aschner M (1996) Astrocytes as modulators of mercury-induced neurotoxicity. Neurotoxicology, **17**: 663–669.

Astic L, Saucier D, Coulon P, Lafay F, & Flamand A (1993) The CVS strain of rabies virus as transneuronal tracer in the olfactory system of mice. Brain Res, **619**: 146–156.

Atterwill CK & Walum E (1989) Neurotoxicology *in vitro*: Model systems and practical applications. Toxicol *In Vitro*, **3**: 159–161.

Audesirk G (1995) Electrophysiological analysis of ion channel function. In: Chang LW & Slikker W ed. Neurotoxicology: Approaches and methods. New York, Academic Press, pp 137–156.

Babich MA (1998) Risk assessment of low-level chemical exposure from consumer products under the U.S. Consumer Product Safety Commission chronic hazard guidelines. Environ Health Perspect, **106**(Suppl 1): 117–120.

Bacon CW, Bennett RM, & Hinton DM (1992) Scanning electron microscopy of *Fusarium moniliforme* within asymptomatic corn kernels and kernels associated with leukoencephalomalacia. Plant Dis, **76**: 144–148.

Baez S, Segura-Aguilar J, Widersten M, Johansson J, & Mannervik R (1997) Glutathione transferases catalyse the detoxication of oxidized metabolites (*o*-quinones) of catecholamines and may serve as an antioxidant system preventing degenerative cellular processes. Biochem J, **324**: 25–28.

Baker H & Spencer RF (1986) Transneuronal transport of peroxidase-conjugated wheat germ agglutinin (WGA-HRP) from the olfactory epithelium to the brain of an adult rat. Exp Brain Res, **63**: 461–473.

Baker EL, Feldman RG, White RA, Harley JP, Niles CA, Dinse GE, Berkey CS (1984) Occupational lead neurotoxicity, a behavioural and electrophysiological evaluation: Study design and year one results. Br J Ind Med, **41**(3): 352–361.

Baker EL, Letz RE, Fidler AT, Shalat S, Plantamura D, & Lyndon M (1985) A computer based neurobehavioural evaluation system for occupational and environmental epidemiology: Methodology and validation studies. Neurobehav Toxicol Teratol, **7**: 369–377.

Balaban CD, O'Callaghan JP, & Billingsley ML (1988) Trimethyltin-induced neuronal damage in the rat brain: Comparative studies using silver degeneration stains, immunocytochemistry and immunoassay for neuronotypic and gliotypic proteins. Neuroscience, **26**(1): 337–361.

Balduini W, Elsner J, Lambardelli G, Peurzzi G, & Cattabeni F (1991) Treatment with methylazoxymethanol at different gestational days: Two way shuttle box avoidance and residential maze activity in rat offspring. Neurotoxicology, **12**: 677–686.

Balin BJ, Broadwell RD, Salcman M, & El-Kalliny M (1986) Avenues for entry of peripherally administered protein to the central nervous system in mouse, rat, and squirrel monkey. J Comp Neurol, 251: 260–280.

Banati RB, Rothe G, Valet G, & Kreutzberg GW (1993) Detection of lysosomal cystein proteinases in microglia: Flow cytometric measurement and histochemical localization of cathepsin B and L. Glia, **7**: 183–191.

Barnes DG & Dourson M (1988) Reference dose (RfD): Description and use in health risk assessments. Regul Toxicol Pharmacol, **8**: 471–486.

Barone S, Stanton ME, & Mundy WR (1995) Neurotoxic effects of neonatal triethyl tin (TET) exposure are exacerbated with aging. Neurobiol Aging, **16**: 723–735.

Becking GC (1995) Use of mechanistic information in risk assessment for toxic chemicals. Toxicol Lett, **77**: 15–24.

Bellinger DC (1995) Interpreting the literature on lead and child development: The neglected role of the "experimental system." Neurotoxicol Teratol, **17**(3): 201–212.

Bellinger DC & Matthews JA (1998) Social and economic dimensions of environmental policy: Lead poisoning as a case study. Perspect Biol Med, **41**(3): 307–326.

Bellinger D, Leviton A, Waterneaux C, Needleman H, & Rabinowitz M (1987) Longitudinal analyses of prenatal and postnatal lead exposure and early cognitive development. N Engl J Med, **316**(17): 1037–1043.

Benignus V (1993) Importance of experimenter-blind procedure in neurotoxicology. Neurotoxicol Teratol, **15**(1): 45–49.

Benveniste EN (1992) Inflammatory cytokines within the central nervous system: Sources, function, and mechanism of action. Am J Physiol, **263**(1 Pt. 1): C1–16.

Bignami A & Dahl D (1976) The astroglial response to stabbing. Immunofluorescence studies with antibodies to astrocyte-specific protein (GFAP) in mammalian and submammalian species. J Neuropathol Appl Neurobiol, **2**: 99–110.

Billmaier D, Yee HT, Allen N, Craft B, Williams N, Epstein S, & Fontaine F (1974) Peripheral neuropathy in a coated fabrics plant. J Occup Med, **16**: 665–671.

Bletner M (1999) Traditional reviews, meta-analyses and pooled analyses in epidemiology. Int J Epidemiol, **28**: 1–9.

Bojic U, Ehlers K, Ellerbeck U, Bacon CL, O'Driscoll E, O'Connell C, Berezin V, Kawa A, Lepekhin E, Bock E, Regan CM, & Nau H (1998) Studies on the teratogen pharmacophore of valproic acid analogues: Evidence of interactions at a hydrophobic centre. Eur J Pharmacol, **354**(2–3): 289–299.

Bolla KI & Roca R (1994) Neuropsychiatric sequelae of occupational exposure to neurotoxins. In: Bleeker ML & Hansen JA ed. Occupational neurology and clinical neurotoxicology. Baltimore, Maryland, Williams and Wilkins, pp 133–158.

Bondy SC (1985) Special considerations for neurotoxicological research. CRC Crit Rev Toxicol, **14**: 381–402.

Bondy SC (1986) The biochemical evaluation of neurotoxic damage. Fundam Appl Toxicol, **6**: 208–216.

Bondy SC (1997) Neurotoxicant-induced oxidative events in the nervous system. In: Lowndes HE & Reuhl KR ed. Comprehensive toxicology. Vol 11. Nervous system and behavioural toxicology. New York, Pergamon Press, pp 59–77.

Bourdiol F, Toulmond S, Serrano A, Benavides J, & Scatton B (1991) Increase in omega 3 (peripheral type benzodiazepine) binding sites in the rat cortex and striatum after local injection of interleukin-1, tumour necrosis factor-alpha and lipopolysaccharide. Brain Res, **543**(3): 194–200.

Bove FJ (1970) The story of ergot. Basel, S. Karger AG.

Bowler RM, Thaler CD, Law D, & Becker CE (1990) Comparison of the NES and CNS/B neuro-psychological screening batteries. Neurotoxicology, **11**(3): 451–464.

Bowler RM, Mergler D, Huel G, Harrison R, & Cone J (1991) Neuropsychological impairment among former microelectronics workers. Neurotoxicology, **12**(1): 87–103.

Boyce S, Kelly E, Reavill C, Jenner P, & Marsen CD (1984) Repeated administration of *N*-methyl-4-phenyl-1,2,5,6-tetrahydropyridine to rats is not toxic to striatal dopamine neurones. Biochem Pharmacol, **33**(11): 1747–1752.

Boyes WK (1992) Testing visual system toxicity using visual evoked potential technology. In: Isaacson RL & Jensen KF ed. The vulnerable brain and environmental risks. Vol. 1. Malnutrition and hazard assessment. New York, Plenum Press, pp 193–222.

Boyes WK (1993) Sensory-evoked potentials: Measures of neurotoxicity. In: Assessing the toxicity of drugs of abuse. Washington, DC, US Department of Health and Human Services, National Institute on Drug Abuse, Alcohol, and Mental Health, pp 63–100 (NIDA Research Monograph 136).

Bradley WG, Daroff RB, Feniehel GM, & Marsden CD ed. (1996) Neurology in clinical practice. Boston, Massachusetts, Butterworth-Heinemann.

Brady ST (1985) A novel brain ATPase with properties expected for the fast axonal transport motor. Nature (Lond), **317**: 73–75.

Brady ST (1991) Molecular motors in the nervous system. Neuron, **7**: 521–533.

Brady S, Lasek R, & Allen R (1985) Video microscopy of fast axonal transport in extruded axoplasm: A new model for study of molecular mechanisms. Cell Motil, **5**(2): 81–101.

Brat DJ & Brimijoin S (1993) Acrylamide and glycidamide impair neurite outgrowth in differentiating N1E.115 neuroblastoma without disturbing rapid bidirectional transport of organelles observed by video microscopy. J Neurochem, **60**(6): 2145–2152.

Brimijoin S & Hammond P (1985) Acrylamide neuropathy in the rat: Effects on energy metabolism in sciatic nerve. Mayo Clin Proc, **60**: 3–8.

Broadwell RD & Balin BJ (1985) Endocytic and exocytic pathways of the neuronal secretory process and trans-synaptic transfer of wheat germ agglutinin-horseradish peroxidase *in vivo*. J Comp Neurol, **242**: 632–650.

Broadwell DK, Darcey DJ, Hudnell HK, Otto DA, & Boyes WK (1995) Work-site clinical and neurobehavioral assessment of solvent-exposed microelectronics workers. Am J Ind Med, **27**: 677–698.

Bruccoleri A, Brown HW, & Harry GJ (1998) Cellular localization and temporal elevation of tumor necrosis factor-alpha, interleukin-1-alpha and transforming growth factor-beta-1 mRNA in hippo-campal injury response induced by trimethyl tin. J Neurochem, **71**: 1577–1587.

Buelke-Sam J, Kimmel CA, & Adams J (1985) Design considerations in screening for behavioural teratogens: Results of the collaborative teratology study. Neurobehav Toxicol Teratol, **7**: 537–589.

Bushnell PJ (1998) Behavioral approaches to the assessment of attention in animals. Psychopharmacology, **138**: 231–259.

Bushnell P, Padilla S, Ward T, Pope C, & Olszyk V (1991) Behavioral and neurochemical changes in rats dosed repeatedly with diisopropylfluorophosphate (DFP). J Pharmacol Exp Ther, **256**: 741–750.

Bushnell PJ, Pope CN, & Padilla S (1993) Behavioural and neurochemical effects of acute chlorpyrifos in rats: Tolerance to prolonged inhibition of cholinesterase. J Pharmacol Exp Ther, **266**(2): 1007–1017.

Caldemeyer KS, Armstrong SW, George KK, Moran CC, & Pascuzzi RM (1996) The spectrum of neuroimaging abnormalities in solvent abuse and their clinical correlation. J Neuroimaging, **6**(3): 167–173.

Caldwell BM & Bradley RH (1984) Home observation for measurement of the environment. Administration manual. Little Rock, Arkansas, University of Arkansas.

Callender TJ, Morrow L, & Subramanian K (1994) Evaluation of chronic neurological sequelae after acute pesticide exposure using SPECT brain scans. J Toxicol Environ Health, **41**: 275–284.

Calne DB, Eisen A, McGeer E, & Spencer PS (1986) Alzheimer's disease, Parkinson's disease, and motoneurone disease: Abiotrophic interaction between ageing and environment? Lancet, **2**(8515): 1067–1070.

Cannon SB, Veazsy JM, Jackson RS, Burse VW, Hayes C, Straub WE, Landrigan PJ, & Liddle JA (1978) Epidemic kepone poisoning in chemical workers. Am J Epidemiol, **107**: 529–537.

Cassells DAK & Dodds EC (1946) Tetra-ethyl lead poisoning. Br Med J, **2**: 4479–4483.

Cassito MG, Gilioli R, & Camerino D (1989) Experiences with the Milan Automated Neurobehavioral System (MANS) in occupational neurotoxic exposures. Neurotoxicol Teratol, **11**: 571–574.

Cavanagh JB, Nolan CC, & Brown AW (1990) Glial cell intrusions actively remove detritus due to toxic chemicals from within nerve cells. Neurotoxicology, **11**: 1–12.

Chang LW (1980) Mercury. In: Spencer PS & Schaumburg HH ed. Experimental and clinical neurotoxicology. Baltimore, Maryland, Williams and Wilkins, pp 508–526.

Chang LW (1995) Neuromorphological and neuropathological approaches. In: Chang LW & Slikker W ed. Neurotoxicology: Approaches and methods. New York, Academic Press, pp 5–27.

Chang LW & Dyer RS ed (1995) Handbook of neurotoxicology. New York, Marcel Dekker.

Chang LW & Verity MA (1995) Mercury neurotoxicity: Effects and mechanisms. In: Chang LW & Dyer RS ed. Handbook of neurotoxicology. New York, Marcel Dekker, pp 31–60.

Chang YC (1987) Neurotoxic effects of n-hexane on the human central nervous system. Evoked potential abnormalities in n-hexane polyneuropathy. J Neurol Neurosurg Psychiatry, **50**: 269–281.

Checkoway H & Cullen MR (1998) Epidemiological methods in occupational neurotoxicology. In: Costa LG & Manzo L ed. Occupational neurotoxicology. Boca Raton, Florida, CRC Press.

Chern CM, Proctor SP, & Feldman RG (1995) Exposure assessment in clinical neurotoxicology: Environmental monitoring and biologic markers. In: Chang LW & Slikker W ed. Neurotoxicology: Approaches and methods. New York, Academic Press, pp 695–709.

Cherry N, Venables H, & Waldron HA (1984) Description of the tests in the London School of Hygiene Test Battery. Scand J Work Environ Health, 10(Suppl): 18–19.

Chia SE, Chia HP, Ong CN, & Jeyaratnam J (1997) Cumulative blood lead levels and neuro-behavioral test performance. Neurotoxicology, 18: 793–803.

Chiba S & Ando K (1976) Effects of chronic administration of kanamycin on conditioned suppression to auditory stimulus in rats. Jpn J Pharmacol, 26(4): 419–426.

Choi DW (1988) Glutamate neurotoxicity and diseases of the nervous system. Neuron, 1: 623–634.

Chouaniere D, Cassitto MG, Spurgeon A, Verdier A, & Gilioli R (1997) An international questionnaire to explore neurotoxic symptoms. Environ Res, 73(1–2): 70–72.

Chu N, Hochberg FH, Calne DB, & Olanow CW (1995) Neurotoxicity of manganese. In: Chang LW & Dyer RS ed. Handbook of neurotoxicology. New York, Marcel Dekker, pp 91–104.

Clark JM (1995) Effects and mechanisms of action of pyrethrin and pyrethroid insecticides. In: Chang LW & Dyer RS ed. Handbook of neurotoxicology. New York, Marcel Dekker, pp 511–546.

Clarke DD & Sokoloff L (1994) Circulation and energy metabolism in the brain. In: Siegal GJ, Agranoff BW, Albers RW, & Molinoff PB ed. Basic neurochemistry. New York, Raven Press, pp 645–680.

Clarke PG & Hornung JP (1989) Changes in the nuclei of dying neurons as studied with thymidine autoradiography. J Comp Neurol, 283(3): 438–449.

Cohn J, Cox C, & Cory-Slechta DA (1993) The effects of lead exposure on learning in a multiple repeated acquisition and performance schedule. Neurotoxicology, 14: 329–346.

Colborn T, vom Saal FS, & Soto AM (1994) Developmental effects of endocrine-disrupting chemicals in wildlife and humans. Environ Health Perspect, 101: 378–384.

Cook DG, Fahn S, & Brait KA (1974) Chronic manganese intoxication. Arch Neurol, 30: 59–71.

Cory-Slechta DA (1989) Behavioural measures of neurotoxicity. Neurotoxicology, 10: 271–296.

Cory-Slechta DA (1990) Bridging experimental animal and human behavioural toxicology studies. In: Russell RW, Flattau PE, & Pope AM ed. Behavioural measures of neurotoxicity. Washington, DC, National Academy Press.

Cory-Slechta DA, Pokora MJ, Fox RA, & O'Mara DJ (1996) Lead-induced changes in dopamine D1 sensitivity: Modulation by drug discrimination training. Neurotoxicology, 17: 445–457.

Cory-Slechta DA & Pounds JG (1995) Lead neurotoxicity. In: Chang LW & Dyer RS ed. Handbook of neurotoxicology. New York, Marcel Dekker, pp 31–60.

Costa LG (1988) Interactions of neurotoxicants with neurotransmitter systems. Toxicology, 49: 359–366.

Costa LG (1996) Biomarker research in neurotoxicology: The role of mechanistic studies to bridge the gap between the laboratory and epidemiological investigations. Environ Health Perspect, **104**(Suppl 1): 55–67.

Costa LG & Manzo L (1998) Biomarkers in occupational neurotoxicology. In: Costa LG & Manzo L ed. Occupational neurotoxicology. Boca Raton, Florida, CRC Press, pp 75–99.

Cotman CW, Gomez-Pinilla F, & Kahle JS (1994) Neuronal plasticity and regeneration. In: Siegal GJ, Agranoff BW, Albers RW, & Molinoff PB ed. Basic neurochemistry. New York, Raven Press, pp 607–626.

Crofton KM (1990) Reflex modification and the detection of toxicant-induced auditory dysfunction. Neurotoxicol Teratol, **12**: 461–468.

Crofton KM, MacPhail RC, & Tilson HA (1996) The use of uncertainty factors in estimating health risks [letter]. Fundam Appl Toxicol, **32**: 126.

Crump KS (1984) A new method for determining allowable daily intakes. Fundam Appl Toxicol, **4**: 854–871.

Cushner IM (1981) Maternal behavior and perinatal risks: Alcohol, smoking, and drugs. Annu Rev Public Health, **2**: 201–218.

Cyr JL & Brady ST (1992) Molecular motors in axonal transport. Cellular and molecular biology of kinesin. Neurobiology, **6**: 137–155.

Damstra T & Bondy SC (1980) The current status and future of biochemical assays for neuro-toxicity. In: Spencer PS & Schaumburg HH ed. Experimental and clinical neurotoxicity. Baltimore, Maryland, Williams and Wilkins, pp 820–833.

Davies PW (1968) The action potential. In: Mountcastle VB ed. Medical physiology, 12th ed. St. Louis, Missouri, C.V. Mosby, pp 1094–1120.

Davis CS & Richardson RJ (1980) Organophosphorous compounds. In: Spencer PS & Schaumburg HH ed. Experimental and clinical neurotoxicology. Baltimore, Maryland, Williams and Wilkins, pp 527–544.

Davis JM & Svendsgaard DJ (1989) U-shaped dose–response curves: Their occurrence and implication for risk assessment. J Toxicol Environ Health, **30**: 71–83.

Dick RB (1988) Short duration exposure to organic solvents: The relationship between neurobehavioural test results and other indicators. Neurotoxicol Teratol, **10**: 35–50.

Dick RB (1995) Neurobehavioral assessment of occupationally relevant solvents and chemicals in humans. In: Chang LW & Dyer RS ed. Handbook of neurotoxicology. New York, Marcel Dekker, pp 217–322.

Dick RB, Bhattacharya A, & Shukla R (1990) Use of a computerized postural sway measurement system for neurobehavioural toxicology. Neurotoxicol Teratol, **12**: 1–6.

Dickson DW, Mattiace LA, Kure K, Hutchins K, Lyman WD, & Bosman CF (1991) Microglia in human disease, with an emphasis on the acquired immune deficiency syndrome. Lab Invest, **64**: 135–156.

Di Monte DA, Royland JE, Irwin I, & Langston JW (1996) Astrocytes as the site for bioactivation of neurotoxins. Neurotoxicology, **17**: 697–703.

Discalzi G, Caparello F, Bottalo L, Fabbro D, & Mocellini A (1993) Auditory brainstem evoked potentials (BAEPs) in lead-exposed workers. Neurotoxicology, **13**: 207–212.

Domjan M & Burkhard B (1986) The principles of learning and memory. Monterey, California, Cole.

Dorman DC, Owens JG, & Morgan KT (1997) Olfactory system. In: Lowndes HE & Reuhl KR ed. Comprehensive toxicology. Vol. 11. Nervous system and behavioural toxicology. New York, Pergamon Press, pp 281–294.

Doull J (1990) Historical perspectives in toxicology. In: Probst GS, Vodicnik MJ, & Dorato MG ed. New horizons in molecular toxicology. Indianapolis, Indiana, Lilly Research Laboratories, pp 5–8.

Durham HD, Dahrouge S, & Cashman S (1993) Evaluation of the spinal cord neuron X neuroblastoma hybrid cell line NSC-34 as a model for neurotoxicity testing. Neurotoxicology, **14**: 387–396.

Dyer RS (1987) Macrophysiological assessment of organometal neurotoxicity. In: Tilson H & Sparber SB ed. Neurotoxicants and neurobiological function. New York, Wiley, pp 137–184.

Dyer RS & Howell WE (1982) Triethyltin: Ambient temperature alters visual system toxicity. Neurobehav Toxicol Teratol, **4**: 267–271.

EC (1996) Technical guidance document in support of commission directive 93/67/EEC on risk assessment for new notified substances and commission regulation EC/1488/94 on risk assessment for existing substances. Luxembourg, European Commission.

EC (1997) Criteria for the qualitative evaluation of human neurobehavioral studies of neurotoxicity. Luxembourg, European Commission, Office for Official Publications of the European Communities.

EC (1999) Report of the Working Group on Endocrine Disrupters of the Scientific Committee on Toxicity, Ecotoxicity and the Environment of DG XXIV (Consumer Policy and Consumer Health Protection). Brussels.

Eccles CU (1988) EEG correlates of neurotoxicity. Neurotoxicol Teratol, **10**: 423–428.

ECETOC (1992) Evaluation of the neurotoxic potential of chemicals. Brussels, European Centre for Ecotoxicology and Toxicology of Chemicals (Monograph No. 18).

ECETOC (1998) Organophosphorous pesticides and long-term effects on the nervous system. Brussels, European Centre for Ecotoxicology and Toxicology of Chemicals (Technical Report No. 75).

ECETOC/UNEP (1996) Inventory of critical reviews on chemicals. Brussels, European Centre for Ecotoxicology and Toxicology of Chemicals; and Geneva, United Nations Environment Programme.

Eckenhoff MF & Rakic P (1991) A quantitative analysis of synaptogenesis in the molecular layer of the dentate gyrus in the rhesus monkey. Brain Res Dev Brain Res, **64**(1–2): 129–135.

Eckerman DA & Bushnell PJ (1992) The neurotoxicology of cognition: Attention, learning and memory. In: Tilson H & Mitchell CL ed. Neurotoxicology. New York, Raven Press, pp 213–270.

Eckerman DA, Caroll JB, Foree D, Gullion CM, Lansman M, Long ER, Waller MB, & Wallsten TS (1985) An approach to brief field testing for neurotoxicity. Neurobehav Toxicol Teratol, 7: 387–393.

Ecobichon DJ & Joy RM (1982) Pesticides and neurologic disease. Boca Raton, Florida, CRC Press.

Eng LF (1985) Glial fibrillary acidic protein (GFAP): The major protein of glial intermediate filaments in differentiated astrocytes. J Neuroimmunol, 8: 203–214.

Eng LF (1988) Astrocytic response to injury. In: Reier PJ, Bunge RP, & Seil FJ ed. Current issues in neural regeneration research. New York, Alan R. Liss, pp 247–255.

Erulkar SD (1994) Chemically mediated synaptic transmission. An overview. In: Siegal GJ, Agranoff BW, Albers RW, & Molinoff PB ed. Basic neurochemistry. New York, Raven Press, pp 181–208.

Escalona E, Yanes L, Feo O, & Maizlish N (1995) Neurobehavioral evaluation of Venezuelan workers exposed to organic solvent mixtures. Am J Ind Med, 27: 15–27.

Evangelista de Duffard A, Bortolozzi A, & Duffard R (1995a) Altered behavioral responses in 2,4-dichlorophenoxyacetic acid treated and amphetamine challenged rats. Neurotoxicology, 16: 479–488.

Evangelista de Duffard AM, Brusco A, Duffard R, Garcia G, & Pecci Saavedra J (1995b) Changes in serotonin-immunoreactivity in the dorsal and median raphe nuclei of rats exposed to 2,4-dichlorophenoxyacetic acid through lactation. Mol Chem Neuropathol, 26: 187–193.

Fechter LD & Young JS (1983) Discrimination of auditory from non-auditory toxicity by reflex modification audiometry: Effects of triethyltin. Toxicol Appl Pharmacol, 70: 216–227.

Fedoroff S & Vernadakis A (1987) Astrocytes. Vol. 2. Orlando, Florida, Academic Press.

Feldman RG (1999) Occupational and environmental neurotoxicology. Philadelphia, Pennsylvania, Lippincott-Raven.

Feldman RG & Ratner MH (1999) The pathogenesis of neurodegenerative disease: Neurotoxic mechanisms of action and genetics. Curr Opin Neurol, 12: 725–731.

Ferri GL, Cichi A, Bastone A, Gaudio RM, Frontali N, & Dahl D (1994) Experimental β,β'-imino-dipropionitrile (IDPN) neuropathy — neurofilament profile of sensory, motor and autonomic nerves as seen by immunocytochemistry on whole-mount preparations. Brain Res, 657: 315–319.

Festing MFW (1991) Genetic factors in neurotoxicology and neuropharmacology: A critical evaluation of the use of genetics as a research tool. Experientia, 12: 1877–1888.

Flegal KM, Keyl PM, & Nieto FJ (1991) Differential misclassification arising from nondifferential errors in exposure measurement. Am J Epidemiol, 134: 1233–1244.

Ford DP, Schwartz BS, & Rothman N (1994) Assessment of exposure and dose in neuro-toxicology: Clinical and epidemiologic applications. In: Bleeker ML & Hansen JA ed. Occupational neurology and clinical neurotoxicology. Baltimore, Maryland, Williams and Wilkins, pp 23–42.

Fowler SC (1987) Force and duration of operant response and dependent variables in behavioural pharmacology. In: Thompson T & Dews PB ed. Advances in behavioural pharmacology. New York, Erlbaum.

FQPA (1996) Food Quality Protection Act. US Congress, Public Law 104-170. Washington, DC, US Government Printing Office.

Frantik E, Hornychova M, & Horvath M (1994) Relative acute neurotoxicity of solvents: Isoeffective air concentration of 48 compounds evaluated in rats and mice. Environ Res, **66**: 173–185.

Frei K, Nadal D, Pfister HW, & Fontana A (1993) Listeria meningitis: Identification of a cerebrospinal fluid inhibitor of macrophage listericidal function as interleukin 10. J Exp Med, **178**(4): 1255–1261.

Fu Y, He F, Zhang S, & Jiao X (1995) Consistent striatal damage in rats induced by 3-nitropropionic acid and cultures of *Arthrinium* fungus. Neurotoxicol Teratol, **17**: 413–418.

Gabbiani G, Gregory A, & Baic D (1967) Cadmium-induced selective lesions of sensory ganglia. J Neuropathol Exp Neurol, **26**: 498–506.

Gad SC (1982) A neuromuscular screen for use in industrial toxicology. J Toxicol Environ Health, **9**: 691, 704.

Gad SC (1989) Principles of screening in toxicology with special emphasis on applications to neurotoxicology. J Am Coll Toxicol, **8**: 21–27.

Gad S & Weil C (1994) Statistics for toxicologists. In: Hayes AW ed. Principles and methods of toxicology, 3rd ed. New York, Raven Press, pp 221–274.

Gade A, Mortensen EL, & Bruhn P (1988) "Chronic painter's syndrome." A reanalysis of psychological test data in a group of diagnosed cases, based on comparisons with matched controls. Acta Neurol Scand, **77**: 293–306.

Gale SD, Hopkins RO, Weaver LK, Bigler ED, Booth EJ, & Blatter DD (1999) MRI, quantitative MRI, SPECT, and neuropsychological findings following carbon monoxide poisoning. Brain Inj, **13**: 229–243.

Gallagher RT, Hawkes AD, Steyn PS, & Vlleggaar R (1984) Tremorgenic neurotoxins from perennial ryegrass causing ryegrass staggers disorders of livestock: Structure and elucidation of Lolitrem. Chem Commun, **18**: 614–616.

Gamberale F, Iregren A, & Kjellberg A (1990) Computerized performance testing in neurotoxicology. Why, what, how and whereto? In: Russel RW, Flattau PE, & Pope AM ed. Behavioral measures of neurotoxicity. Washington, DC, National Academy Press, pp 359–395.

Garner JA (1988) Differential turnover of tubulin and neurofilaments in central nervous system neuron terminals. Brain Res, **458**: 309–318.

Gaylor DW & Slikker W Jr (1990) Risk assessment for neurotoxic effects. Neurotoxicology, **11**: 211–218.

Gaylor DW & Slikker W (1996) Reply to Re: The use of uncertainty factors in estimating health risks [letter]. Fundam Appl Toxicol, **32**: 127.

Gebicke-Haerter PJ, VanCalker D, Norenberg W, & Illes P (1996) Molecular mechanisms of microglial activation. Implications for regeneration and neurodegenerative diseases. Neurochem Int, **29**: 1–12.

Gehrmann J, Matsumoto Y, & Kreutzberg GW (1995) Microglia: Intrinsic immuneffector cell of the brain. Brain Res Rev, **20**: 269–287.

Gerr F & Letz R (1988) Reliability of a widely used test of peripheral cutaneous vibration sensitivity and a comparison of two testing protocols. Br J Ind Med, **45**: 635–639.

Gerr F & Letz R (1993) Vibrotactile threshold testing in occupational health: A review of current issues and limitations. Environ Res, **60**: 145–159.

Gerr F, Hershman D, & Letz R (1990) Vibrotactile threshold measurement for detecting neurotoxicity: Reliability and determination of age- and height-standardized normative values. Arch Environ Health, **45**: 148–154.

Ghantous H, Dencker L, Gabrielsson J, Danielsson BR, & Bergman K (1990) Accumulation and turnover of metabolites of toluene and xylene in nasal mucosa and olfactory bulb in the mouse. Pharmacol Toxicol, **66**: 87–92.

Gibson JL (1904) A plea for painted railings and painted walls of rooms as the source of lead poisoning amongst Queensland children. Aust Med Gaz, **23**: 149.

Gilbert ME & Burdette LJ (1995) Hippocampal field potentials: A model system to characterize neurotoxicity. In: Chang LW & Slikker W ed. Neurotoxicology: Approaches and methods. New York, Academic Press, pp 183–204.

Giulian D (1993) Reactive glia as rivals in regulating neuronal survival. Glia, **7**: 102–110.

Giulian D & Vaca K (1993) Inflammatory glia mediate delayed neuronal damage after ischemia in the CNS. Stroke, **24**: 184–190.

Giulian D, Chen J, Ingeman JE, George JK, & Noponen M (1989) The role of mononuclear phagocytes in wound healing after traumatic injury to adult mammalian brain. J Neurosci, **9**(12): 4416–4429.

Giulian D, Li L, Li X, George J, & Rutecki PA (1994) The impact of microglia-derived cytokines upon gliosis in the CNS. Dev Neurosci, **16**: 128–136.

Glasgow HB, Burkholder JM, Schmechel DE, Tester PA, & Rublee PA (1995) Insidious effects of a toxic estuarine dinoflagellate on fish survival and human health. J Toxicol Environ Health, **46**: 501–522.

Glowa JR (1991) Dose–effect approaches to risk assessment. Neurosci Biobehav Rev, **15**: 153–158.

Glowa JR & MacPhail RC (1995) Qualitative approaches to risk assessment in neurotoxicology. In: Chang LW & Slikker W ed. Neurotoxicology: Approaches and methods. New York, Academic Press, pp 777–787.

Gobba F, Galassi C, Imbiani M, Ghittori S, Candea S, & Cavalleri A (1991) Acquired dys-chromatopsia among styrene-exposed workers. J Occup Med, **33**: 761–765.

Goetz CG (1985) Pesticides and other environmental toxins. In: Neurotoxins in clinical practice. New York, Spectrum Publications, Inc., pp 107–131.

Goldberg AM & Frazier JM (1989) Alternatives to animals in toxicity testing. Sci Am, **261**: 24–30.

Golden PL & Pardridge WM (2000) Brain microvascular P-glycoprotein and a revised model of multidrug resistance in brain. Cell Mol Neurobiol, **20**(2): 165–181.

Goldey ES & Crofton KM (1998) Thyroxine replacement attenuates hypothyroxinemia, hearing loss, and motor deficits following developmental exposure to Aroclor 1254 in rats. Toxicol Sci, **45**(1): 94–105.

Goldmuntz EA, Brosnan CF, Chiu FC, & Norton WT (1986) Astrocytic reactivity and intermediate filament metabolism in experimental autoimmune encephalomyelitis: The effect of suppression with prazosin. Brain Res, **397**: 16–26.

Goldstein MK & Stein GH (1985) Ambulatory activity in chronic disease. In: Tryon WH ed. Behavioural assessment in behavioural medicine. New York, Springer Publishing Co., pp 160–162.

Goldsworthy TL, Recio L, Brown K, Donehower LA, Mirsalis JC, Tennant RW, & Purchase IFH (1994) Transgenic animals in toxicology. Fundam Appl Toxicol, **22**: 8–19.

Gonzalez MF, Shiraish K, Hissanga K, Sagar SM, Mandabach M, & Sharp FR (1989) Heat shock proteins as marker of neural injury. Mol Brain Res, **6**: 93–100.

Graeter LJ & Mortenson ME (1996) Kids are different: Developmental variability in toxicology. Toxicology, **111**: 15–20.

GrandPre T, Nakamura F, Vartanian T, & Strittmatter SM (2000) Identification of the Nogo inhibitor of axon regeneration as a Reticulon protein. Nature, **403**: 439–444.

Griffin JW (1990) Basic pathologic processes in the nervous system. Toxicol Pathol, **18**: 83–88.

Guyot MC, Hantraye P, Dolan R, Palfi S, Maziere R (1997) Quantifiable bradykinesia, gait abnormalities and Huntington's disease-like striatal lesions in rats chronically treated with 3-nitropropionic acid. Neuroscience, **79**: 45–56.

Hageman G, van der Hoek J, van Hout M, van der Laan G, Steur EJ, de Bruin W, & Herholz K (1999) Parkinsonism, pyramidal signs, polyneuropathy, and cognitive decline after long-term occupational solvent exposure. J Neurol, **246**: 198–206.

Hammerschlag R & Stone GC (1982) Membrane delivery by fast axonal transport. Trends Neurosci, **5**: 12–15.

Hammerschlag R, Cyr JL, & Brady S (1994) Axonal transport and the neuronal cytoskeleton. In: Siegal GJ, Agranoff BW, Albers RW, & Molinoff PB ed. Basic neurochemistry. New York, Raven Press, pp 545–572.

Hänninen H (1971) Psychological picture of manifest and latent carbon disulfide poisoning. Br J Ind Med, **28**: 374–381.

Hänninen H (1990a) Methods in behavioural toxicology: Current test batteries and need for development. In: Russell RW, Flattau PE, & Pope AM ed. Behavioural measures of neurotoxicity. Washington, DC, National Academy Press.

Hänninen H (1990b) The neuropsychological screening test battery: Validation and current uses in Finland. In: Johnson BL, Anger WK, Durao A, & Xintaras C ed. Advances in neurobehavioural toxicology: Applications in environmental and occupational health. Chelsea, Michigan, Lewis Publishers, pp 257–262.

Hansch C & Kim D (1989) Toward a quantitative comparative toxicology of organic compounds. Crit Rev Toxicol, **19**: 185–226.

Hany J, Lilienthal H, Sarasin A, Roth-Harer A, Fastabend A, Dunemann L, Lichtensteiger W, & Winneke G (1999) Developmental exposure of rats to a reconstituted PCB mixture or Aroclor 1254: Effects on organ weights, aromatase activity, sex hormone levels, and sweet preference behavior. Toxicol Appl Pharmacol, **158**(3): 231–243.

Harry GJ (1992) Acrylamide-induced alterations in axonal transport. Biochemical and autoradiographic studies. Mol Neurobiol, **6**: 203–216.

Harry GJ ed (1994) Development neurotoxicology. Boca Raton, Florida, CRC Press, p 177.

Harry GJ (1999) Basic principles of disturbed CNS and PNS functions. In: Niesink RJM, Jaspers RMA, Kornet LMW, van Ree JM, & Tilson HA ed. Introduction to neurobehavioral toxicology: Food and environment. Boca Raton, Florida, CRC Press, pp 115–162.

Harry GJ & Bruccoleri A (1999) Neuroimmunotoxicology. In: Tilson H & Harry GJ ed. Neurotoxicology. New York, Taylor and Francis, pp 219–264.

Harry GJ, Morell P, & Bouldin TW (1992) Acrylamide exposure preferentially impairs axonal transport of glycoproteins in myelinated axons. J Neurosci Res, **31**: 554–560.

Harry GJ, Billingsley M, Bruinink A, Campbell IL, Classen W, Dorman DC, Galli C, Ray D, Smith RA, & Tilson HA (1998) In vitro techniques for the assessment of neurotoxicity. Environ Health Perspect, **106**: 131–158.

Hartman DE (1988) Neuropsychological toxicology: Identification and assessment of human neurotoxic syndromes, 1st ed. New York, Pergamon Press.

Hartman DE (1995) Neuropsychological toxicology: Identification and assessment of human neurotoxic syndromes, 2nd ed. New York, Plenum Press.

Hastings L (1990) Sensory neurotoxicology. Use of the olfactory system in the assessment of toxicity. Neurotoxicol Teratol, **12**: 455–459.

Hauser SL, Doolittle TH, Lincoln R, Brown RH, Dialrello CA (1990) Cytokine accumulations in CSF of multiple sclerosis patients: Frequent detection of interleukin-1 and tumor necrosis factor but not interleukin-6. Neurology, **40**: 1735–1739.

Hayes WJ (1991) Studies in humans. In: Hayes W & Lawes ER ed. Handbook of pesticide toxicology. San Diego, California, Academic Press, pp 215–244.

He F (1985) Occupational toxic neuropathies — An update. Scand J Work Environ Health, **11**: 321–330.

He F, Zhang S, Wang H, Li G, Zhang Z, Li F, Dong X, & Hu F (1989) Neurological and electro-neuromyographic assessment of the adverse effects of acrylamide on occupationally exposed workers. Scand J Work Environ Health, **15**: 125–129.

He F, Zhang S, & Zhang C (1990) Mycotoxin induced encephalopathy and dystonia in children. In: Volans GN, Sims J, Sullivan FM, & Turner P ed. Basic science in toxicology. London, Taylor & Francis, p 596.

He F, Zhang S, Qian F, & Zhang C (1995) Delayed dystonia with striatal CT lucencies induced by a mycotoxin (3-nitropropionic acid). Neurology, **45**: 2178–2183.

Health Canada (1994) Human health risk assessment for Priority Substances. Ottawa, Health Canada, Environmental Health Directorate (Publication No. En40-215/41E).

Heikkila RE, Hess A, & Duvoisin RC (1984) Dopaminergic neurotoxicity of 1-methyl-4-phenyl-1,2,5,6-tetrahydropyridine in mice. Science, **224**: 1451–1453.

Heise GA (1984) Behavioural methods for measuring effects of drugs on learning and memory in animals. Med Res Rev, **4**: 535–558.

Herr D & Boyes W (1995) Electrophysiological analysis of complex brain systems: Sensory evoked potentials and their generators. In: Chang LW & Slikker W ed. Neurotoxicology: Approaches and methods. New York, Academic Press, pp 205–224.

Hertel RF (1996) Outline on risk assessment of existing substances in the European Union. Environ Toxicol Pharmacol, **2**: 93–96.

Heuser G & Mena I (1994) NeuroSPECT findings in patients exposed to neurotoxic chemicals. Toxicol Ind Health, **10**: 561–571.

Hill AB (1965) The environment and disease: Association or causation? Proc R Soc Med, **58**: 295–300.

Hill RM & Tennyson LM (1986) Maternal drug therapy: Effect on fetal and neonatal growth and neurobehavior. Neurotoxicology, **7**: 121–140.

Hille B & Catterall WA (1994) Electrical excitability and ion channels. In: Siegal GJ, Agranoff BW, Albers RW, & Molinoff PB ed. Basic neurochemistry. New York, Raven Press, pp 75–96.

Hogstedt C, Andersson K, & Hane M (1984) A questionnaire approach to the monitoring of early disturbances in central nervous function. In: Aito A, Rihimäki V, & Vainio H ed. The biological monitoring of exposure to industrial chemicals. Washington, DC, Hemisphere, pp 275–287.

Holtmaat AJGD, Oestreicher AB, Gispen WH, & Verhaagen J (1998) Manipulation of gene expression in the mammalian nervous system. Application in the study of neurite outgrowth and neuroregeneration-related proteins. Brain Res Rev, **26**: 43–71.

Hooisma J, Emmen HH, Kulig BM, Muijser H, Poortvliet D, & Letz R (1990) Factor analysis of tests from the Neurobehavioural Evaluation System and the WHO Neurobehavioural Core Test Battery. In: Johnson B, Anger WK, Durao A, & Xintaras C ed. Advances in neurobehavioural toxicology: Applications in environmental and occupational health. Chelsea, Michigan, Lewis Publishers, pp 245–256.

Hooisma J, Hänninen H, Emmen HH, & Kulig BM (1994) Symptoms indicative of the effects of organic solvent exposure in Dutch painters. Neurotoxicol Teratol, 16: 613–622.

Horan JM, Kurt TL, Landrigan PJ, Melius M, & Singal M (1985) Neurologic dysfunction from exposure to 2-*t*-butylazo-2-hydroxy-5-methylhexane (BHMH): A new occupational neuropathy. Am J Public Health, 75: 513–517.

Hruska RE, Kennedy S, & Silbergeld EK (1979) Quantitative aspects of normal locomotion in rats. Life Sci, 25: 171–179.

Hudnell HK, Otto DA, & House DE (1996) The influence of vision on computerized neuro-behavioral test scores: A proposal for improving test protocols. Neurotoxicol Teratol, 18: 391–400.

Hughes JA & Sparber SB (1978) d-Amphetamine unmasks postnatal consequences of exposure to methylmercury *in utero*: Methods for studying behavioral teratogenesis. Pharmacol Biochem Behav, 8: 365–375.

IARC (1987) Overall evaluations of carcinogenicity: An updating of IARC monographs volumes 1 to 42. Lyon, International Agency for Research on Cancer (IARC Monographs on the Evaluation of Carcinogenic Risks to Humans, Suppl 7).

ICME (1994) A guide to neurotoxicity: International regulation and testing strategies. Ottawa, International Council on Metals and the Environment.

Ikonomidou C, Bittigau P, Ishimaru MJ, Wozniak DF, Koch C, Genz K, Price MT, Stefovska V, Horster F, Tenkova T, Dikranian K, Olney JW (2000) Ethanol-induced apoptotic neurodegeneration and fetal alcohol syndrome. Science, 287: 1056–1060.

IPCS (1983) Environmental health criteria 27: Guidelines on studies in environmental epidemiology. Geneva, World Health Organization, International Programme on Chemical Safety.

IPCS (1984) Environmental health criteria 30: Principles for evaluating health risks to progeny associated with exposure to chemicals during pregnancy. Geneva, World Health Organization, International Programme on Chemical Safety.

IPCS (1986a) Environmental health criteria 59: Principles for evaluating health risks from chemicals during infancy and early childhood. Geneva, World Health Organization, International Programme on Chemical Safety.

IPCS (1986b) Environmental health criteria 60: Principles and methods for the assessment of neurotoxicity associated with exposure to chemicals. Geneva, World Health Organization, International Programme on Chemical Safety.

IPCS (1987) Environmental health criteria 70: Principles for the safety assessment of food additives and contaminants in food. Geneva, World Health Organization, International Programme on Chemical Safety.

IPCS (1992) Environmental health criteria 144: Principles for evaluating the effects of chemicals on the aged population. Geneva, World Health Organization, International Programme on Chemical Safety.

IPCS (1993) Environmental health criteria 155: Biomarkers and risk assessment. Geneva, World Health Organization, International Programme on Chemical Safety.

IPCS (1994) Environmental health criteria 170: Assessing human health risks of chemicals: derivation of guidance values for health-based exposure limits. Geneva, World Health Organization, International Programme on Chemical Safety.

IPCS (1996a) Environmental health criteria 180: Principles and methods for the assessment of immunotoxicity associated with exposures to chemicals. Geneva, World Health Organization, International Programme on Chemical Safety.

IPCS (1996b) Environmental health criteria 187: White spirit. Geneva, World Health Organization, International Programme on Chemical Safety.

IPCS (1999) Environmental health criteria 210: Principles for the assessment of risks to human health from exposure to chemicals. Geneva, World Health Organization, International Programme on Chemical Safety.

Iregren A (1998) Computer-assisted testing. In: Costa LG & Manzo L ed. Occupational neurotoxicology. Boca Raton, Florida, CRC Press, pp 213–233.

IUPAC (1998) Natural and anthropogenic environmental oestrogens. International Union of Pure and Applied Chemistry. Pure Appl Chem, **70**(9): 1617–1865.

Jabre JF (1995) Electrophysiological investigations of toxic neuropathies. In: Chang LW & Slikker W ed. Neurotoxicology: Approaches and methods. New York, Academic Press, pp 737–745.

Jacobson JL & Jacobson SW (1996) Intellectual impairment in children exposed to polychlorinated biphenyls *in utero*. N Engl J Med, **335**: 783–789.

Jacobson JL & Jacobson SW (1999) Assessing neurotoxicity in children. In: Tilson HA & Harry GJ ed. Neurotoxicology. New York, Taylor and Francis, pp 339–366.

Jacobson M (1991) Developmental neurobiology. New York, Plenum Press.

Jacobson SW, Fein GG, Jacobson JL, Schwartz PM, & Dowler JK (1985) The effect of intrauterine PCB exposure on visual recognition memory. Child Dev, **56**: 853–860.

Jarabek AM, Menache MG, Overton JH, Dourson ML, & Miller FJ (1990) The US Environmental Protection Agency's inhalation RfD methodology: Risk assessment for air toxics. Toxicol Ind Health, **6**: 279–301.

Jeppson R (1975) Parabolic relationship between lipophilicity and biological activity of aliphatic hydrocarbons, ethers and ketones after intravenous injection of emulsion formulation into mice. Acta Pharmacol Toxicol, **37**: 56–64.

Johnsen H, Lund SP, Matikainen E, Midtgard U, Simonsen L, & Wennberg A (1992) Occupational neurotoxicity: Criteria document for evaluation of existing data. Copenhagen, Nordic Council of Ministers and National Institute of Occupational Health.

Johnson MK (1988) Sensitivity and selectivity of compounds interacting with neuropathy target esterase: Further structure–activity studies. Biochem Pharmacol, **37**: 4095–4104.

Johnson BL, Baker EL, El Batawi M, Gilioli R, Hänninen H, Seppäläinen AM, & Xintaras C (1987) Prevention of neurotoxic illness in working populations. New York, John Wiley & Sons.

Johnson MK (1990) Organophosphates and delayed neuropathy. Is NTE alive and well? Toxicol Appl Pharmacol, **102**: 385–399.

Jonkman EJ, De Weerd AW, Poorttvliet DCJ, Veldhuizen RJ, & Emmen H (1992) Electroencephalographic studies in workers exposed to solvents and pesticides. Electroencephalogr Clin Neurophysiol, **82**: 438–444.

Joy RM, Stark LG, & Albertson TE (1982) Proconvulsant effects of lindane: Enhancement of amygdaloid kindling in the rat. Neurobehav Toxicol Teratol, **4**: 347–354.

Joyner AL & Guillemont F (1994) Gene targeting and development of the nervous system. Curr Opin Neurobiol, **4**: 37–42.

Kavlock RJ, Daston GP, DeRosa C, Fenner-Crisp P, Gray LE, Kaatten S, Lucier G, Luster M, Mac M, Maczka C, Miller R, Moore J, Rolland R, Scott G, Sheehan DM, Sinks T, & Tilson HA (1996) Research needs for assessment of health and environmental effects of endocrine disruptors: A report of the US EPA sponsored workshop. Environ Health Perspect, **104**: 715–740.

Kelly RB (1985) Pathways of protein secretion in eukaryotes. Science, **230**: 25–32.

Kieswetter E, Sietmann B, & Seeber A (1997) Standardization of a questionnaire for neurotoxic symptoms. Environ Res, **73**: 73–80.

Kimmel CA (1988) Current status of behavioural teratology: Science and regulation. CRC Crit Rev Toxicol, **19**: 1–10.

Kimmel CA & Buelke-Sam J ed. (1994) Developmental toxicology, 2nd ed. New York, Raven Press, pp 429–453.

Kimmel CA & Kimmel GL (1996) Principles of developmental toxicology risk assessment. In: Hood RD ed. Handbook of developmental toxicology. Boca Raton, Florida, CRC Press, pp 667–693.

Kimmel CA, Rees DC, & Francis EZ (1990) Qualitative and quantitative comparability of human and animal developmental neurotoxicology. Teratology, **12**: 175–292.

Kimmel CA, Kavlock RF, & Francis EZ (1992) Animal models for assessing developmental toxicity. In: Guzelian PS, Henry CJ, & Olin SS ed. Similarities and differences between children and adults: Implications for risk assessment. Washington, DC, ILSI Press, pp 43–65.

King RHM (1999) Atlas of peripheral nerve pathology. London, Arnold.

Kipen HM & Fiedler N (1999) Invited commentary: Sensitivities to chemicals — context and implications. Am J Epidemiol, **150**: 13–16.

Klaassen CD (1982) Neurotoxic lesions of cadmium in young rats. Toxicol Appl Pharmacol, **63**: 330–337.

Klaassen CD, Amdur MO, & Doull J ed. (1986) Casarett and Doull's toxicology: The basic science of poisons, 3rd ed. New York, Macmillan.

Klaassen CD, Amdur MO, & Doull J ed. (1996) Casarett and Doull's toxicology: The basic science of poisons, 5th ed. New York, McGraw-Hill.

Kopin IJ & Markey SP (1988) MPTP toxicity: Implications for research in Parkinson's disease. Annu Rev Neurosci, **11**: 81–96.

Kotsonis FN & Klaassen CD (1977) Toxicity and distributions of cadmium administered to rats at sublethal doses. Toxicol Appl Pharmacol, **41**: 667–680.

Kreutzberg GW (1987) Microglia. In: Adelman G ed. Encyclopedia of neuroscience. Boston, Massachusetts, Birkhauser, pp 661–662.

Kreutzberg GW (1996) Microglia: A sensor for pathological events in the CNS. Trends Neurosci, **19**(8): 312–328.

Krinke GJ (1989) Neuropathologic screening in rodent and other species. J Am Coll Toxicol, **8**: 141–155.

Krishnan K & Andersen ME (1994) Physiologically based pharmacokinetic modeling in toxicology. In: Hayes AW ed. Principles and methods in toxicology, 3rd ed. New York, Raven Press, pp 149–188.

Kristersson K (1987) Retrograde transport of macromolecules in axons. Annu Rev Pharmacol Toxicol, **18**: 91–110.

Kukull WA, Larson EB, Bowen JD, McCormick WC, Teri L, Pfanschmidt ML, Thompson JD, O'Meara ES, Brenner DE, & Van Bell G (1995) Solvent exposure as a risk factor for Alzheimer's disease: A case–control study. Am J Epidemiol, **141**: 1059–1071.

Kulig BM (1996) Comprehensive neurotoxicity assessment. Environ Health Perspect 1990; **104**(Suppl 2): 317–322.

Kulig B, Alleva E, Bignami G, Cohn J, Cory-Slechta D, Landa V, O'Donoghue J, & Peakall D (1996) Animal behavioral methods in neurotoxicity assessment: SGOMSEC joint report. Environ Health Perspect, **104**(Suppl 2): 193–204.

Kurata H (1990) Mycotoxins and mycotoxicoses: Overview. In: Pohland AE, Dowell VR Jr, & Richards JL ed. Microbial toxins in foods and feeds, cellular and molecular modes of action. New York, Plenum Press, pp 249–259.

Ladefoged O, Lam HR, Ostergaard G, & Nielsen E (1995) Neurotoxicology: Review of definitions, methodology and criteria. Copenhagen, National Food Agency of Denmark and Danish Environmental Protection Agency (Miljoprojeckt nr. 282).

Lai JCK, Guest G, Haglid KG, Rosengren L, Porcellati G, & Kjellstrand P (1980) The effects of cadmium, manganese and aluminum on sodium-potassium-activated and magnesium-activated adenosine triphosphatase activity and choline uptake in rat brain synaptosomes. Biochem Pharmacol, **29**: 41–49.

Landauer MR, Tomlinson NT, Balster RL, & MacPhail RC (1984) Some effects of the formamidine pesticide chlordimeform on the behavior of mice. Neurotoxicology, **5**: 91–100.

Landrigan PJ, Graham DG, & Thomas RD (1994) Environmental neurotoxic illness: Research for prevention. Environ Health Perspect, **102**(Suppl 2): 117–120.

Landrigan PJ, Weiss B, Goldman LR, Carpenter DO, & Suk WA ed (2000) The developing brain and the environment. Environ Health Perspect **108**(Suppl 3): 373–595.

Langston JW, Ballard P, Tetrud JW, & Irwin I (1983) Chronic parkinsonism in humans due to a product of meperidine-analog synthesis. Science, **219**: 979–980.

Lasek RJ & Brady ST (1982) The structural hypothesis of axonal transport: Two classes of moving elements. In: Weiss DG ed. Axoplasmic transport. Berlin, Springer-Verlag, pp 397–405.

Lasek RJ, Garner J, & Brady S (1984) Axonal transport of the cytoplasmic matrix. J Cell Biol, **99**: 212s–221s.

Lassmann H, Zimprich F, Vass K, & Hickey WF (1991) Microglial cells are a component of the perivascular glia limitans. J Neurosci Res, **28**: 236–243.

Last JM (1986) Epidemiology and health information. In: Last JM ed. Maxcy-Rosenau public health and preventive medicine. New York, Appleton-Century-Crofts.

Laursen P (1990) A computer-aided technique for testing cognitive functions validated on a sample of Danes 30 to 60 years of age. Acta Neurol Scand Suppl, **131**: 1–108.

Lawson LJ, Perry VH, Dri P, & Gordon S (1990) Heterogeneity in the distribution and morphology of microglia in the normal adult mouse brain. Neuroscience, **39**: 151–170.

LeBel CP & Foss JA (1996) Use of a rodent neurotoxicity screening battery in preclinical safety assessment of recombinant-methionyl human brain-derived neurotrophic factor. Neurotoxicology, **17**(3–4): 851–863.

LeBel CP, Ali SF, McKee M, & Bondy SC (1990) Organometal-induced increases in oxygen radical activity: The potential of 2',7'-dichlorofluorescin diacetate as an index of neurotoxic damage. Toxicol Appl Pharmacol, **104**: 17–28.

Lee MH & Rabe A (1992) Premature decline in Morris water maze performance of aging micrencephalic rats. Neurotoxicol Teratol, **14**(6): 383–392.

Lehman AJ & Fitzhugh OG (1954) 100-fold margin of safety. US Q Bull, **18**: 33–35.

Letz R (1991) Use of computerized test batteries for quantifying neurobehavioral outcomes. Environ Health Perspect, **90**: 195–198.

Letz R (1993) Covariates of computerized neurobehavioral test performance in epidemiologic investigations. Environ Res, **61**: 124–132.

Lewis JL, Hahn FF, & Dahl AR (1994) Transport of inhaled toxicants to the central nervous system. Characteristics of a nose–brain barrier. In: Isaacson RL & Jensen KF ed. The vulnerable brain and environmental risks. Vol. 3. New York, Plenum Press, pp 77–103.

Lezak MD (1983) Neuropsychological assessment, 2nd ed. New York, Oxford University Press.

Li AA (1994) The use (misuse) of schedule-controlled operant behavior in neurotoxicity testing. In: Weiss B & O'Donoghue J ed. Neurobehavioral toxicity: Analysis and interpretation. New York, Raven Press, pp 243–252.

Lilienthal H & Winneke G (1991) Sensitive periods for behavioural toxicity of polychlorinated biphenyls: Determination by cross-fostering in rats. Fundam Appl Toxicol, **17**: 368–375.

Lipton SA (1992) Models of neuronal injury in AIDS: Another role for the NMDA receptor? Trends Neurosci, **15**: 75–79.

London L, Myers JE, Nell V, Taylor T, & Thompson ML (1997) An investigation into neurologic and neurobehavioral effects of long-term agrichemical use among deciduous fruit farm workers in the Western Cape, South Africa. Environ Res, **73**: 132–145.

Longstreth WT, Koepsell TD, & Van Belle G (1994) Neuroepidemiology as it applies to occupational neurology. In: Bleeker ML & Hansen JA ed. Occupational neurology and clinical neurotoxicology. Baltimore, Maryland, Williams and Wilkins, pp 1–21.

Lotti M (1995) Mechanisms of toxicity and risk assessment. Toxicol Lett, **77**: 9–14.

Ludolph AC & Spencer PS (1995) Mycotoxins and tremorogens: Effects and mechanisms. In: Chang LW & Dyer RS ed. Handbook of neurotoxicology. New York, Marcel Dekker, pp 591–610.

Lundberg I, Hogberg M, Michélsen H, Nise G, & Hogsted C (1997) Evaluation of the Q16 questionnaire on neurotoxic symptoms and a review of its use. Occup Environ Med, **54**: 343–350.

Lundh B, Love A, Kristensson K, & Norrby E (1988) Non-lethal infection of aminergic reticular core neurones: Age-dependent spread of ts mutant vesicular stomatitis virus from the nose. J Neuropathol Exp Neurol, **47**: 497–506.

MacPhail RC (1985) Effects of pesticides on schedule-controlled behavior. In: Seiden LS & Balster RL ed. Behavioural pharmacology: The current status. New York, Alan R. Liss, pp 519–535.

MacPhail RC (1990) Environmental modulation of neurotoxicity. In: Russell RW, Flattau PE, & Pope AM ed. Behavioural measures of neurotoxicity. Washington, DC, National Academy Press.

MacPhail RC, Crofton KM, & Reiter LW (1983) Use of environmental challenges in behavioural toxicology. Fed Proc, **42**: 3196–3200.

MacPhail RC, Peele DB, & Crofton KM (1989) Motor activity and screening for neurotoxicity. J Am Coll Toxicol, **8**: 117–125.

MacPhail RC, Tilson HA, Mose VC, Becking GC, Cuomo V, Frantik E, Kulig BM, & Winneke G (1997) The IPCS collaborative study on neurobehavioral screening methods: Background and genesis. Neurotoxicology, **18**: 925–928.

MacTutus CF, Unger KL, & Tilson HA (1982) Neonatal chlordecone exposure impairs early learning and memory in the rat on a multiple measure passive avoidance task. Neurotoxicology, **3**: 27–44.

Mailman RB (1987) Mechanisms of CNS injury in behavioural dysfunction. Neurotoxicol Teratol, **9**: 417–426.

Malecki EA, Cook BM, Devenyi AG, Beard JL, & Connor JR (1999) Transferrin is required for normal distribution of ^{59}Fe and ^{54}Mn in mouse brain. J Neurol Sci, 170: 112–118.

Manzo L, Artigas F, Martinez R, Mutti A, Bergamaschi E, Nicotera P, Tonini M, Candura SM, Ray DE, & Costa LG (1996) Biochemical markers of neurotoxicity: A review of mechanistic studies and applications. Hum Exp Toxicol, **15**(Suppl 1): S20–S35.

Maroni M & Catenacci G (1994) Biological monitoring of neurotoxic compounds. In: Bleeker ML & Hansen JA ed. Occupational neurology and clinical neurotoxicology. Baltimore, Maryland, Williams and Wilkins, pp 43–89.

Martenson CH, Odom A, Sheetz MP, & Graham DG (1995) The effect of acrylamide and other sulfhydryl alkylators on the ability of dynein and kinesin to translocate microtubules *in vitro*. Toxicol Appl Pharmacol, **133**(1): 73–81.

Martin-Bouyer G, Lebreton R, Toga M, Stolley PD, & Lockhart J (1982) Outbreak of accidental hexachlorophene poisoning in France. Lancet 1(8263): 91–95.

Matthews HB, Dixon D, Herr DW, & Tilson HA (1990) Subchronic toxicity studies indicate that tris(2-chloroethyl)phosphate administration results in lesions in the rat hippocampus. Toxicol Ind Health, **6**: 1–15.

Mattsson JL & Albee RR (1988) Sensory evoked potentials in neurotoxicology. Neurotoxicol Teratol, **10**: 435–443.

Mattsson MP, Barger SW, Furukawa K, Bruce AJ, Wyss-Coray T, Mark RJ, & Mucke L (1997) Cellular signaling roles of TGF beta, TNF alpha and beta APP in brain injury responses and Alzheimer's disease. Brain Res Rev, **23**: 47–61.

Maurissen JP (1988) Quantitative sensory assessment in toxicology and occupational medicine: Applications, theory and critical appraisal. Toxicol Lett, **43**: 321–343.

Maurissen JP (1995) Neurobehavioural methods for the evaluation of sensory functions. In: Chang LW & Slikker W ed. Neurotoxicology: Approaches and methods. New York, Academic Press, pp 239–264.

Maurissen JP, Weiss B, & Davis HT (1983) Somatosensory thresholds in monkeys exposed to acrylamide. Toxicol Appl Pharmacol, **71**: 266–279.

Maxwell DM, Lenz DE, Croff WA, Kaminskis A, & Froehlich HL (1987) The effects of blood flow and detoxification on *in vivo* cholinesterase inhibition by Soman in rats. Toxicol Appl Pharmacol, **88**: 66–76.

McEwen B (1994) Endocrine effects on the brain and their relationship to behavior. In: Siegal GJ, Agranoff BW, Albers RW, & Molinoff PB ed. Basic neurochemistry. New York, Raven Press, pp 1003–1023.

McMartin DN, O'Donoghue JL, Morrissey R, & Fix AS (1997) Non-proliferative lesions of the nervous system in rats. In: Guides for toxicologic pathology. Woodbury, New Jersey, Society for Toxicologic Pathology.

McMillan DE & Owens SM (1995) Extrapolating scientific data from animals to humans in behavioural toxicology and behavioural pharmacology. In: Chang LW & Slikker W ed. Neurotoxicology: Approaches and methods. New York, Academic Press, pp 323–332.

Mehta PS, Bruccoleri A, Brown HW, & Harry GJ (1998) Increase in brain stem cytokine mRNA levels as an early response to chemical-induced myelin edema. J Neuroimmunol, **88**: 154–164.

Mergler D (1995) Behavioural neurophysiology: Quantitative measures of sensory function. In: Chang LW & Slikker W ed. Neurotoxicology: Approaches and methods. New York, Academic Press, pp 727–736.

Mergler D, Huel G, Belanger S, Bowler RM, Truchon G, Drolet D, & Ostiguy C (1996) Surveillance of early neurotoxic dysfunction. Neurotoxicology, **17**: 803–812.

Merigan WH (1979) Effects of toxicants on visual systems. Neurobehav Toxicol, **1**(Suppl 1): 15–22.

Metcalf RL (1995) Carbamate and thiocarbamate neurotoxicity. In: Chang LW & Dyer RS ed. Handbook of neurotoxicology. New York, Marcel Dekker, pp 547–556.

Mikkelsen S (1995) Solvent encephalopathy: Disability pension studies and other case studies. In: Chang LW & Dyer RS ed. Handbook of neurotoxicology. New York, Marcel Dekker, pp 323–338.

Misson JP, Takahishi T, & Caviness VS (1991) Ontogeny of radial and other astroglial cells in murine cerebral cortex. Glia, **4**: 138–148.

Mitchell JD & Shaw IC (1999) Natural food factors. In: Niesink RJM, Jaspers RMA, Kornet LMW, van Ree JM, & Tilson HA ed. Introduction to neurobehavioral toxicology. Food and environment. Boca Raton, Florida, CRC Press, pp 230–251.

Morata TC & Dunn DE (1994) Occupational exposure to noise and ototoxic organic solvents. Arch Environ Health, **49**: 359–365.

Morell P & Mailman RB (1987) Selective and nonselective effects of organometals on brain neurochemistry. In: Tilson HA & Sparber SB ed. Neurotoxicants and neurobiological function: Effects of organoheavy metals. New York, Wiley, pp 201–230.

Morrison SJ (1999) Prospective identification, isolation by flow cytometry, and *in vivo* self-renewal of multipotent mammalian neural crest cells. Cell, **96**: 737–749.

Moser VC (1989) Screening approaches to neurotoxicity: A functional observational battery. J Am Coll Toxicol, **8**: 85–93.

Moser VC (1995) Comparisons of the acute effects of cholinesterase inhibitors using a neuro-behavioural screening battery in rats. Neurotoxicol Teratol, **17**: 617–625.

Moser VC (1997) Behavioural screening for neurotoxicity. In: Lowndes HE & Reuhl KR ed. Comprehensive toxicology. Vol. 11. Nervous system and behavioural toxicology. New York, Pergamon Press, pp 351–362.

Moser VC, McDaniel KL, & Phillips PM (1991) Rat strain and stock comparisons using a functional observational battery: Baseline values and effects of amitraz. Toxicol Appl Pharmacol, **108**: 267–283.

Muhammad BY & Kitchen I (1994) Effect of chronic maternal diazepam treatment on the development of stress-induced antinociception in young rats. Pharmacol Biochem Behav, **47**: 927–933.

Muijser H, Hooisma J, Hoogendijk EM, & Twisk DA (1986) Vibration sensitivity as a parameter for detecting peripheral neuropathy. I. Results in healthy workers. Int Arch Environ Occup Health, **58**: 287–299.

Murthy RT, Saxena DK, Sunderman V, & Chandra SV (1987) Cadmium-induced ultrastructural changes in the cerebellum of weaned and adult rats. Ind Health, **25**: 159–162.

Mutti A & Smargiassi A (1998) Selective vulnerability of dopaminergic systems to industrial chemicals: Risk assessment of related neuroendocrine changes. Toxicol Ind Health, **14**(1–2): 311–323.

Myers GJ & Davidson PW (1998) Prenatal methylmercury exposure and children: Neurologic, developmental, and behavioral research. Environ Health Perspect, **106**(Suppl 3): 841–847.

Nagymajtenyi L, Schulz H, & Desi I (1995) Changes in EEG of freely-moving rats caused by three-generation organophosphate treatment. Arch Toxicol Suppl, **17**: 288–294.

Needleman HL (1987) Introduction: Biomarkers in neurodevelopmental toxicology. Environ Health Perspect, **74**: 149–152.

Needleman HL (1990) Lessons from the history of childhood plumbism for pediatric neuro-toxicology. In: Johnson BL, Anger WK, Durano A, & Xintaras C ed. Advances in neurobehavioural toxicology: Applications in experimental and occupational health. Chelsea, Michigan, Lewis Publishers, pp 331–337.

Needleman HL, Gunnoe CE, & Leviton A (1979a) Deficits in psychologic and classroom performance of children with elevated blood lead levels. N Engl J Med, **300**: 695–702.

Needleman HL, Gunnoe C, Leviton LA, Reed R, Peresie H, Maher C, & Barret P (1979b) Deficits in psychologic and classroom performance with elevated dentin lead levels. N Engl J Med, **300**: 689–695.

Needleman HL, Schell A, Bellinger D, Leviton A, & Alfred EN (1990) The long-term effects of exposure to low doses of lead in childhood: An 11 year follow-up report. N Engl J Med, **322**(2): 83–88.

Needleman HL, Riess JA, Tobin MJ, Bieseker GE, & Greenhouse JB (1996) Bone lead levels and delinquent behaviour. J Am Med Assoc, **275**: 363–369.

Nelson BK (1986) Behavioral teratology of industrial solvents. In: Riley EP & Vorhees CV ed. Handbook of behavioural teratology. New York, Plenum Press, pp 391–406.

Nelson BK (1991a) Evidence for behavioural teratogenicity in humans. J Appl Toxicol, **11**: 33–37.

Nelson BK (1991b) Selecting exposure parameters in developmental neurotoxicity assessments. Neurotoxicol Teratol, **13**: 569–573.

Nelson K, Golnick J, Korn T, & Angle C (1993) Manganese encephalopathy: Utility of early magnetic resonance imaging. Br J Ind Med, **50**(6): 510–513.

Neuwelt EA (1989) Implication of the blood–brain barrier and its manipulation. New York, Plenum Medical.

Newland MC (1988) Quantification of motor function in toxicology. Toxicol Lett, **43**: 295–319.

Newland MC (1995) Motor functions and the physical properties of the operant: Applications to screening and advanced techniques. In: Chang LW & Slikker W ed. Neurotoxicology: Approaches and methods. New York, Academic Press, pp 265–299.

Newland MC (1997) Neural, behavioural and measurement considerations in the detection of motor impairment. In: Lowndes HE & Reuhl KR ed. Comprehensive toxicology. New York, Pergamon Press, pp 309–331.

Nicotera P, Leist M, & Ferrando-May E (1998) Intracellular ATP, a switch in the decision between apoptosis and necrosis. Toxicol Lett, **103**: 139–142.

Nies KJ & Sweet JJ (1994) Neuropsychological assessment and malingering: A critical review of past and present strategies. Arch Clin Neuropsychol, **9**: 501–552.

Nishino H, Kumazaki M, Fukuda A, Fujimoto I, Shimano Y, Hida H, Sakurai T, Deshpande SB, Shimizu H, Morikawa S, & Inubushi T (1997) Acute 3-nitroproprionic acid intoxication induces striatal astrocytic cell death and dysfunction of the blood–brain barrier: Involvement of dopamine toxicity. Neurosci Res, **27**: 343–355.

Norton WT & Cammer W (1984) Chemical pathology of diseases involving myelin. In: Morrel P ed. Myelin. New York, Plenum Press, pp 311–335.

Nuwer M (1997) Assessment of digital EEG, quantitative EEG, and EEG brain mapping: Report of the American Academy of Neurology and the American Clinical Neurophysiology Society. Neurology, **49**(1): 277–292.

O'Callaghan JP (1988) Neurotypic and gliotypic proteins as biochemical markers of neurotoxicity. Neurotoxicol Teratol, **10**: 445–452.

Ochs S (1987) The action of neurotoxins in relation to axoplasmic transport. Neurotoxicology, **8**: 155–166.

O'Donoghue JL (1989) Screening for neurotoxicity using a neurologically based examination and neuropathology. J Am Coll Toxicol, **8**: 97–116.

O'Donoghue JL (1994) Defining what is neurotoxic. In: Weiss B & O'Donoghue JL ed. Neuro-behavioural toxicity: Analysis and interpretation. New York, Raven Press, pp 19–33.

OECD (1981) Test Guidelines 1981. Acute inhalation toxicity (TG403). Paris, Organisation for Economic Co-operation and Development.

OECD (1987a) Test Guidelines 1987. Acute dermal toxicity (TG402). Paris, Organisation for Economic Co-operation and Development.

OECD (1987b) Test Guidelines 1987. Acute eye irritation/corrosion (TG405). Paris, Organisation for Economic Co-operation and Development.

OECD (1992) Test Guidelines 1992. Acute oral toxicity — fixed dose method (TG420). Paris, Organisation for Economic Co-operation and Development.

OECD (1995) Test Guidelines 1995. Delayed neurotoxicity of organophosphorus substances following acute exposure (TG418) and 28-day repeated dose study (TG419). Paris, Organisation for Economic Co-operation and Development.

OECD (1996) Test Guidelines 1996. Acute oral toxicity — acute toxic class method (TG423). Paris, Organisation for Economic Co-operation and Development.

OECD (1997) Test Guidelines 1997. Neurotoxicity study in rodents (TG424). Paris, Organisation for Economic Co-operation and Development.

OECD (1998) Test Guidelines 1998. Repeated dose 90-day oral toxicity study in rodents (TG408). Paris, Organisation for Economic Co-operation and Development.

OECD (1999) Draft Test Guidelines 1999. Developmental neurotoxicity study (TG426). Paris, Organisation for Economic Co-operation and Development.

OECD/IPCS (2001) Project on the harmonization of chemical hazard/risk assessment terminology: Critical analysis of survey results. Organisation for Economic Co-operation and Development and World Health Organization, International Programme on Chemical Safety (in press).

Otis JA & Handler JS (1995) Evoked potential testing in clinical neurotoxicology. In: Chang LW & Slikker W ed. Neurotoxicology: Approaches and methods. New York, Academic Press, pp 747–751.

Ott L, McClain CJ, Gilespie M, & Young B (1995) Cytokines and metabolic dysfunction after severe head injury. J Neurotrauma, **11**: 447–472.

Otto DA & Hudnell HK (1990) Electrophysiological systems for neurotoxicity field testing: PEARL II and alternatives. In: Johnson B, Anger WK, Durao A, & Xintaras C ed. Advances in neuro-behavioural toxicology: Applications in environmental and occupational health. Chelsea, Michigan, Lewis Publishers, pp 259–276.

Otto DA & Hudnell HK (1993) The use of visual and chemosensory evoked potentials in environmental and occupational health. Environ Res, **62**: 159–171.

Padilla S, Wilson VZ, & Bushnell PJ (1994) Studies on the correlation between blood cholines-terase inhibition and "tissue" inhibition in pesticide-treated rats. Toxicology, **92**: 11–25.

Pardridge W (1998) Introduction to blood–brain barrier. Cambridge, Cambridge University Press.

Paule MG, Forrester TM, Maher MA, Cranmer JM, & Allen RR (1990) Monkey versus human performance in the NCTR operant test battery. Neurotoxicol Teratol, **12**: 503–507.

Pearson DT & Dietrich KN (1985) The behavioral toxicology and teratology of childhood: Models, methods, and implications for intervention. Neurotoxicology, **6**: 165–182.

Peele DB & Vincent A (1989) Strategies for assessing learning and memory, 1978–1987: A comparison of behavioural toxicology, psychopharmacology and neurobiology. Neurosci Biobehav Rev, **13**: 33–38.

Peele DB, Allison SD, & Crofton KM (1990) Learning and memory deficits in rats following exposure to 3,3'-iminodipropionitrile. Toxicol Appl Pharmacol, **105**: 321–332.

Pentreath VW ed (1999) Neurotoxicology *in vitro*. London, Taylor and Francis.

Perl TM, Bedard L, Kosatsky T, Hockin JC, Todd ECD, & Remis RS (1990) An outbreak of toxic encephalopathy caused by eating mussels contaminated with domoic acid. N Engl J Med, **322**: 1775–1780.

Perry JH & Liebelt RA (1961) Extra-hypothalamic lesions associated with gold-thioglucose induced obesity. Proc Soc Exp Biol Med, **106**: 55–57.

Perry VH, Andersson PB, & Gordon S (1993) Macrophages and inflammation in the central nervous system. Trends Neurosci, **16**: 268–273.

Peters A, Palay SL, & Webster H (1991) The fine structure of the nervous system. Neurons and their supporting cells, 3rd ed. New York, Oxford University Press.

Pierce PE, Thompson JF, Hikaskey WH, Nickey LN, Barthel WF, & Hinman AR (1972) Alkyl mercury poisoning in humans. Report of an outbreak. J Am Med Assoc, **220**: 1439–1442.

Plato N & Steineck G (1993) Methodology and utility of a job-exposure matrix. Am J Ind Med, **23**: 491–502.

Pocock SJ, Smith M, & Baghurst P (1994) Environmental lead and children's intelligence: A systematic review of the epidemiological literature. Br Med J, **309**: 1189–1197.

Politis MJ, Schaumburg HH, & Spencer PS (1980) Neurotoxicity of selected chemicals. In: Spencer PS & Schaumburg HH ed. Experimental and clinical neurotoxicology. Baltimore, Williams and Wilkins, pp 613–630.

Porterfield S (1994) Vulnerability of the developing brain to thyroid abnormalities: Environmental insults to the thyroid system. Environ Health Perspect, **102**: 125–130.

Prichep LS & John ER (1992) QEEG profiles of psychiatric disorders. Brain Topogr, **4**: 249–257.

Prockop LD (1995) Neuroimaging in neurotoxicology. In: Chang LW & Slikker W ed. Neurotoxicology: Approaches and methods. New York, Academic Press, pp 753–763.

Prockop LD & Naidu KA (1999) Brain CT and MRI findings after carbon monoxide toxicity. J Neuroimaging, **9**(3): 175–181.

Pryor G, Dickinson J, Howd RA, & Rebert CS (1983) Transient cognitive deficits and high-frequency hearing loss in weanling rats exposed to toluene. Neurobehav Toxicol Teratol, **5**: 53–57.

Radatz M, Ehlers K, Yagen B, Bialer M, & Nau H (1998) Alnoctamide, valpromide and valnoctic acid are much less teratogenic in mice than valproic acid. Epilepsy Res, **30**: 41–48.

Raine CS (1994) Neurocellular anatomy. In: Siegal GJ, Agranoff BW, Albers RW, & Molinoff PB ed. Basic neurochemistry. New York, Raven Press, pp 3–32.

Raitta C, Seppäläinen AM, & Huuskonen MS (1978) *n*-Hexane maculopathy in industrial workers. Albrecht Von Graefes Arch Klin Exp Ophthalmol, **209**(2): 99–110.

Rakic P (1971) Guidance of neurons migrating to the fetal monkey neocortex. Brain Res, **33**: 471–476.

Rakic P (1972) Mode of cell migration to the superficial layers of fetal monkey neocortex. J Comp Neurol, **145**: 61–84.

Rao BL & Husain A (1985) Presence of cyclopiazonic acid in Kodo millet (*Paspalum scrobiculatum*) causing "Kodua poisoning" in man and its production by associated fungi. Mycopathologia, **89**: 177–180.

Ray DE (1997) Function in neurotoxicity: Index of effect and also determinant of vulnerability. Clin Exp Pharmacol Physiol, **24**: 857–860.

Ray DE (1999a) Chronic effects of low level exposure to anticholinesterases — a mechanistic review. Toxicol Lett, **103**: 527–533.

Ray DE (1999b) 3-Nitropropionic acid (NPA). In: Bondy SC ed. Advances in neurodegenerative disorders. Scottsdale, Arizona, Prominent Press, pp 132–159.

Rebert CS (1983) Multisensory evoked potentials in experimental and applied neurotoxicology. Neurobehav Toxicol Teratol, **5**: 659–671.

Rees DC & Hattis D (1994) Developing quantitative strategies for animal to human extrapolation. In: Hayes AW ed. Principles and methods of toxicology. New York, Raven Press, pp 275–315.

Renwick AG & Lazarus NR (1998) Human variability and noncancer risk assessment: An analysis of the default uncertainty factor. Regul Toxicol Pharmacol, **30**: 3–20.

Reuhl KR (1991) Delayed expression of neurotoxicity: The problem of silent damage. Neurotoxicology, **12**: 341–346.

Rice DC (1988) Quantification of operant behavior. Toxicol Lett, **43**: 361–379.

Rice DC & Karpinski KF (1988) Lifetime low-level lead exposure produces deficits in delayed alternation in adult monkeys. Neurotoxicol Teratol, **10**: 207–214.

Richardson RJ (1995) Assessment of the neurotoxic potential of chlorpyrifos relative to other organophosphorous compounds: A critical review of the literature. J Toxicol Environ Health, **44**: 135–165.

Riepe MW, Hori N, Ludolph AC, & Carpenter DO (1995) Failure of neuronal ion exchange, not potentiated excitation, causes excitotoxicity after inhibition of oxidative phosphorylation. Neuroscience, **64**(1): 91–97.

Riley AL & Tuck DL (1985) Conditioned taste aversions: A behavioural index of toxicity. Ann NY Acad Sci, **443**: 272–292.

Riley EP & Vorhees CV ed (1986) Handbook of behavioural teratology. New York, Plenum Press.

Ritter S & Dinh TT (1988) Capsaicin-induced neuronal degeneration: Silver impregnation of cell bodies, axons, and terminals in the central nervous system of the adult rat. J Comp Neurol, **271**(1): 79–90.

Robbins MS, Hughes JA, Sparber SB, & Mannering GJ (1978) Delayed teratogenic effects of methylmercury on hepatic cytochrome P-450 dependent monooxygenase systems of rats. Life Sci, **4**: 287–294.

Robbins TW, Muir JL, Killcross AS, & Pretsell D (1993) Methods for assessing attention and stimulus control. In: Sahgal A ed. Behavioural neuroscience. Vol. 1. A practical approach. New York, IRL Press, pp 13–47.

Rodier PM (1986) Time of exposure and time of testing in developmental neurotoxicology. Neurotoxicology, **7**: 69–76.

Rodier P (1990) Developmental neurotoxicology. Toxicol Pathol, **18**: 89–95.

Romero I, Brown AW, Cavanagh JB, Nolan CC, Ray DE, & Seville MP (1991) Vascular factors in the neurotoxic damage caused by 1,3-dinitrobenzene in the rat. Neuropathol Appl Neurobiol, **17**: 495–508.

Rosenberg NL (1995) Basic principles of clinical neurotoxicology. In: Chang LW & Slikker W ed. Neurotoxicology: Approaches and methods. New York, Academic Press, pp 617–627.

Rosner D & Markowitz G (1985) A "gift of God"? The public health controversy over leaded gasoline during the 1920s. Am J Public Health, **75**: 344–352.

Ross JF & Lawhorn GT (1990) ZPT-related distal axonopathy: Behavioral and electrophysiologic correlates in rats. Neurotoxicol Teratol, **12**(2): 153–159.

Ross JF, Broadwell RD, Poston MR, & Lawhorn GT (1994) Highest brain bismuth levels and neuropathology are adjacent to fenestrated blood vessels in mouse brain after intraperitoneal dosing of bismuth subnitrate. Toxicol Appl Pharmacol, **124**: 191–200.

Ross JF, Switzer RC, Poston MR, & Lawhorn GT (1996) Distribution of bismuth in the brain after intraperitoneal dosing of bismuth subnitrate in mice: Implications for routes of entry of xenobiotic metals into the brain. Brain Res, **725**: 137–154.

Rothman KJ ed (1988) Causal inference. Chestnut Hill, Massachusetts, Epidemiology Resources Inc.

Rothman KJ & Greenland S (1998) Modern epidemiology, 2nd ed. New York, Lippincott Williams & Wilkins.

Ruijten MWMM, Sallé HJA, Verberk MM, & Muijser H (1990) Special nerve functions and color discrimination in workers with long-term low level exposure to carbon disulphide. Br J Ind Med, **47**: 589–595.

Ruijten MWMM, Hooisma J, Brons JT, Habets CEP, Emmen HH, & Muijser H (1994) Neuro-behavioral effects of long-term exposure to xylene and mixed organic solvents in shipyard spray painters. Neurotoxicology, **15**(3): 613–620.

Russell RW (1991) Essential roles for animal models in understanding human toxicities. Neurosci Biobehav Rev, **15**: 7–11.

Ryan CM, Morrow LA, Bromet EJ, & Parkinson DK (1987) Assessment of neuropsychological dysfunction in the workplace: Normative data from the Pittsburgh Occupational Exposures Test Battery. J Clin Exp Neuropsychol, **9**: 665–679.

Sabri MI (1986) Chemical neurotoxins and disruptions of the axonal transport system. In: Iqbal Z ed. Axoplasmic transport. Boca Raton, Florida, CRC Press, pp 185–208.

Sahenk Z & Lasek RJ (1988) Inhibition of proteolysis blocks anterograde-retrograde conversion of axonally transported vesicles. Brain Res, **460**: 199–203.

Sakane T, Akizuki M, Yamashita S, Nada T, Hashida M, & Sezaki H (1991) The transport of a drug to the cerebrospinal fluid directly from the nasal cavity: The relation to the lipophilicity of the drug. Chem Pharm Bull, **39**: 2456–2458.

Saneto RP & deVellis J (1987) Neuronal and glial cells: Cell culture of the central nervous system. In: Turner AJ & Bachelard HS ed. Neurochemistry — A practical approach. Washington, DC, IRL Press, pp 27–63.

Sanz P, Flores IC, Soriano T, Repetto G, Repetto M (1995) *In vitro* quantitative structure–activity relationship assessment of pyrrole adducts production by gamma-diketone-forming neurotoxic solvents. Toxicol *In Vitro*, 9: 783–787.

Scallet AC (1995) Quantitative morphometry for neurotoxicity assessment. In: Chang LW & Slikker W ed. Neurotoxicology: Approaches and methods. New York, Academic Press, pp 99–132.

Schantz SL, Levin ED, Bowman RE, Heironimus MP, & Laughlin NK (1989) Effects of perinatal PCB exposure on discrimination-reversal learning in monkeys. Neurotoxicol Teratol, 11: 243–250.

Schaumburg HH (2000) Human neurotoxic disease. In: Spencer PS, Schaumburg HH, & Ludolph AC ed. Experimental and clinical neurotoxicology. New York, Oxford University Press, pp 55–82.

Schiønning JD (1993) Retrograde transport of mercury in rat sciatic nerve. Toxicol Appl Pharmacol, 121: 43–49.

Schmued LC & Hopkins KJ (2000) Fluoro-Jade: Novel fluorochromes for detecting toxicant-induced neuronal degeneration. Toxicol Pathol, 28(1): 91–99.

Schrot J, Thomas JR, & Robertson RF (1984) Temporal changes in repeated acquisition behavior after carbon monoxide exposure. Neurobehav Toxicol Teratol, 6: 23–28.

Seeber A, Blaszkewicz, Golka K, & Kieswetter E (1997) Solvent exposure and ratings of well-being: Dose–effect relationships and consistency of data. Environ Res, 73: 81–91.

Selmaj KW, Farooq M, Norton WT, Raine CS, Brosnan CF (1990) Proliferation of astrocytes *in vitro* in response to cytokines. A primary role for tumor necrosis factor. J Immunol, 144: 129–135.

Seppäläinen AM (1988) Neurophysiological approaches to the detection of early neurotoxicity in humans. CRC Crit Rev Toxicol, 18: 245–298.

Seppäläinen AM (1998) Electrophysiological approaches to occupational neurotoxicology. In: Costa LG & Manzo L ed. Occupational neurotoxicology. Boca Raton, Florida, CRC Press, pp 185–197.

Seppäläinen AM & Haltia M (1980) Carbon disulfide. In: Spencer PS & Schaumburg HH ed. Experimental and clinical neurotoxicology. Baltimore, Maryland, Williams and Wilkins, pp 356–373.

Sette WR (1994) The role of schedule-controlled operant behavior in the identification of toxic effects of environmental chemicals. In: Weiss B & O'Donoghue ed. Neurobehavioral toxicity: Analysis and interpretation. New York, Raven Press, pp 231–241.

Sette WF & MacPhail RC (1992) Qualitative and quantitative issues in assessment of neurotoxic effects. In: Tilson H & Mitchell C ed. Neurotoxicology. New York, Raven Press, pp 345–361.

SGOMSEC (1996) Risk assessment for neurobehavioural toxicity. Scientific Group on Methodologies for the Safety Evaluation of Chemicals. Environ Health Perspect, 104(Suppl 4): 171–412.

Shafer TJ (1999) The role of ion channels in neurotoxicity. In: Tilson HA & Harry GW ed. Neurotoxicology. New York, Taylor and Francis, pp 99–137.

Shafer TJ & Atchison WD (1995) Electrophysiological methods for analysis of effects of neurotoxicants on synaptic transmission. In: Chang LW & Slikker W ed. Neurotoxicology: Approaches and methods. New York, Academic Press, pp 157–182.

Shahar A, deVellis J, Vernadakis A, & Haber B (1989) A dissection and tissue culture manual of the nervous system. New York, Alan R. Liss, Inc.

Shaughnessy LW, Barone S, Mundy WR, Herr DW, & Tilson HA (1994) Comparison of intracranial infusions of colchicine and ibotenic acid as models of neurodegeneration in the basal forebrain. Brain Res, **637**: 15–26.

Sheng JG, Mrak RE, & Griffin WS (1995) Microglial interleukin-1 alpha expression in brain regions in Alzheimer's disease: Correlation with neuritic plaque distribution. Neuropathol Appl Neurobiol, **21**: 290–301.

Shipley M (1985) Transport of molecules from nose to brain: Transneuronal anterograde and retrograde labeling in the rat olfactory system by wheat germ agglutinin-horseradish peroxidase applied to the nasal epithelium. Brain Res Bull, **15**: 129–142.

Sickles DW, Brady ST, Testino A, Friedman MA, & Wrenn RW (1996) Direct effect of the neurotoxicant acrylamide on kinesis-based microtubule motility. J Neurosci Res, **46**: 7–17.

Silbergeld EK (1987) Neurochemical approaches to developing markers of neurotoxicity: Review of current status and evaluation of future prospects. Environ Res, **63**: 274–286.

Simonsen L, Midtgard U, Lund SP, & Hass U (1995) Occupational neurotoxicity: Evaluation of neurotoxicity data for selected chemicals. Copenhagen, Nordic Council of Ministers.

Simpson LL, Considine RV, Coffied JA, Jeyapaul J, & Bakry NM (1995) Bacterial toxins that act on the nervous system. In: Chang LW & Dyer RS ed. Handbook of neurotoxicology. New York, Marcel Dekker, pp 563–589.

Slikker W (1997) The developing nervous system. In: Lowndes HE & Reuhl KR eds. Comprehensive toxicology. Vol. 11. Nervous system and behavioural toxicology. New York, Pergamon Press, pp 295–308.

Slikker W, Crump KS, Andersen ME, & Bellinge D (1996) Biologically based, quantitative risk assessment of neurotoxicants. Fundam Appl Toxicol, **29**: 18–30.

Slob W & Pieters MN (1998) A probabilistic approach for deriving acceptable human intake limits and human health risks from toxicological studies: General framework. Risk Anal, **18**: 787–798.

Smargiassi A, Bergamaschi E, Mutti A, & Cella MT (1998) Predictive validity of the Q16 questionnaire: A comparison between reported symptoms and neurobehavioral tests. Neurotoxicology, **19**: 703–708.

Smith MA, Grant LD, & Sors AI ed (1989) Lead exposure and child development: An international assessment. Dordrecht, Kluwer Academic Publishers.

Sobotka TJ, Ekelman KB, Slikker W Jr, Raffaele K, & Hattan DG (1996) Food and Drug Administration proposed guidelines for neurotoxicological testing of food chemicals. Neurotoxicology, **17**: 825–836.

Spencer PS & Schaumburg HH ed (1980) Experimental and clinical neurotoxicology. Baltimore, Maryland, Williams and Wilkins.

Spencer PS & Schaumburg HH (1985) Organic solvent neurotoxicity. Facts and research needs [review]. Scand J Work Environ Health, **11**(Suppl 1): 53–60.

Spencer PS, Sabri MI, Schaumburg HH, & Moore CL (1979) Does a defect of energy metabolism in the nerve fiber underlie axonal degeneration in polyneuropathies? Ann Neurol, **5**(6): 501–507.

Spencer PS, Miller MS, Ross SM, Schwab B, Sabri MI (1987a) Biochemical mechanisms underlying primary degeneration in axons. In: Laijth S ed. Handbook of neurochemistry. New York, Plenum Press, pp 155–166.

Spencer PS, Nunn PB, Hugon J, Ludolph AC, Ross SM, Roy DN, & Robertson RC (1987b) Guam amyotrophic lateral sclerosis–Parkinsonism–dementia linked to a plant excitant neurotoxin. Science, **237**: 517–522.

Spencer PS, McCauley LA, Joos SK, Lasarev MR, Schuell T, Bourdette D, Barkhuizen A, Johnston W, Storzbach D, Wynn M, & Grewenow R (1998) U.S. Gulf War veterans: Service periods in theater, differential exposures, and persistent unexplained illness. Toxicol Lett, **102–103**: 515–521.

Spencer PS, Schaumburg HH, & Ludolph AC ed (2000) Experimental and clinical neurotoxicology, 6th ed. New York, Oxford University Press.

Spreafico R, De Biasi S, Frassoni C, & Battaglia G (1985) Transneuronal transport of wheatgerm agglutinin conjugated with horseradish peroxidase in the somatosensory system of the rat: A light- and electron-microscopic study. Somatosens Res, **3**: 119–137.

Spyker JM (1975) Assessing the impact of low level chemicals on development. Behavioral and latent effects. Fed Proc, **34**: 1835–1844.

Squibb RE, Tilson HA, Meyer OA, & Lamartiniere CA (1981) Neonatal exposure to monosodium glutamate alters the neurobehavioral performance of adult rats. Neurotoxicology, **2**(3): 471–484.

Stanton ME & Freeman JH (1994) Eye-blink conditioning in the infant rat: An animal model of learning and developmental neurotoxicology. Environ Health Perspect, **102**: 131–139.

Stanton ME & Spear LP (1990) Comparability of endpoints across species in developmental neurotoxicity. Neurotoxicol Teratol, **12**: 261–268.

Steinhauer SR, Morrow LA, Condray R, & Dougherty GG (1997) Event-related potentials in workers with ongoing occupational exposure. Biol Psychiatry, **42**(9): 854–858.

Stephens R & Barker P (1998) Role of human neurobehavioral tests in regulatory activity on chemicals. Occup Environ Med, **55**: 210–214.

Steventon G, Waring RH, Sturman S, Heafield MT, & Williams AC (1999) Metabolism of S-carboxymethyl-L-cysteine in humans: A neurodegenerative disease study. Med Sci Res, **27**: 119–120.

Stewart P (1999) Exposure assessment in community-based epidemiological studies. Lancet, **353**(9167): 1816–1817.

Stokes WS & Marafante E (1998) Introduction and summary of the thirteenth meeting of the Scientific Group on Methodologies for the Safety Evaluation of Chemicals: Alternative testing methodologies. Environ Health Perspect, **106**(Suppl 2): 405–412.

Streit WJ, Graeber MF, & Kreutzberg GW (1988) Functional plasticity of microglia: A review. Glia, **1**: 301–307.

Struve FA, Straumanis JJ, & Patrick G (1994) Persistent topographic quantitative EEG sequelae of chronic marijuana use: A replication study and initial discriminant analysis. Clin Electro-encephalogr, **25**: 63–75.

Sullivan E, Rosenbloom M, & Pfefferbaum A (1998) Effect of neurotoxins revealed through *in vivo* brain imaging. In: Tilson H & Harry G ed. Neurotoxicology. New York, Taylor and Francis, pp 287–309.

Suzuki K (1980) Special vulnerabilities of the developing nervous system to toxic substances. In: Spencer PS & Schaumburg HH ed. Experimental and clinical neurotoxicology. Baltimore, Maryland, Williams and Wilkins, pp 48–61.

Switzer RC (2000) Application of silver degeneration stains for neurotoxicity testing. Toxicol Pathol, **28**: 70–83.

Tandon P, Padilla S, Barone S, Pope CN, & Tilson HA (1994) Fenthion produces a persistent decrease in muscarinic receptor function in the adult rat retina. Toxicol Appl Pharmacol, **125**: 271–280.

Thompson FN Jr & Porter JK (1990) Tall fescue toxicosis in cattle: Could there be a public health problem. Vet Hum Toxicol, **32**: 51–57.

Thuomas KA, Moller C, Odkvist LM, Flodin U, & Dige N (1996) MR imaging in solvent-induced chronic toxic encephalopathy. Acta Radiol, **37**: 177–179.

Tielemans E, Heederik D, Burdorf A, Vermeulen R, Veulemans G, Kromhout H, & Hartog K (1999) Assessment of occupational exposures in a general population: Comparisons of different methods. Occup Environ Med, **56**: 145–151.

Tilson HA (1990a) Behavioural indices of neurotoxicity. Toxicol Pathol, **18**: 96–104.

Tilson HA (1990b) Neurotoxicology in the 1990s. Neurotoxicol Teratol, **12**: 293–300.

Tilson HA (1997) Learning and memory. In: Lowndes HE & Reuhl KR ed. Nervous system and behavioural toxicology. New York, Pergamon Press, pp 379–390.

Tilson HA (1998a) The concern for developmental neurotoxicology: Is it justified and what is being done about it? Environ Health Perspect, **103**: 147–151.

Tilson HA (1998b) Developmental neurotoxicology of endocrine disruptors and pesticides: Identification of information gaps and research needs. Environ Health Perspect, **106**(Suppl 3): 807–811.

Tilson HA & Cabe PA (1978) Strategy for the assessment of neurobehavioural consequences of environmental factors. Environ Health Perspect, 26: 287–299.

Tilson HA & Mitchell CL (1983) Neurotoxicants and adaptive responses of the nervous system. Fed Proc, **42**: 3189–3190.

Tilson HA & Mitchell CL (1984) Neurobehavioural techniques to assess the effects of chemicals on the nervous system. Annu Rev Pharmacol Toxicol, **24**: 25–50.

Tilson HA & Moser VC (1992) Comparison of screening approaches. Neurotoxicology, **13**: 1–14.

Tilson HA, Squibb RE, Meyer OA, & Sparber SB (1980) Postnatal exposure to benzene alters the neurobehavioural functioning of rats when tested during adulthood. Neurobehav Toxicol Teratol, **2**: 101–106.

Tilson HA, Shaw S, & McLamb RL (1987) The effects of lindane, DDT, and chlordecone on avoidance responding and seizure activity. Toxicol Appl Pharmacol, **88**: 57–65.

Tilson HA, MacPhail RC, & Crofton KM (1995) Defining neurotoxicity in a decision-making context. Neurotoxicology, **16**: 363–376.

Tilson HA, MacPhail RC, & Crofton KM (1996) Setting exposure standards: A decision process. Environ Health Perspect, **104**: 401–405.

Tilson HA, MacPhail RC, Moser VC, Becking GC, Cuomo V, Frantik E, Kulig BM, & Winneke G (1997) The IPCS collaborative study on neurobehavioural screening methods: VII. Summary and conclusions. Neurotoxicology, **18**: 1065–1070.

Toews AD & Morell P (1999) Molecular biological approaches in neurotoxicology. In: Tilson HA, & Harry GJ ed. Neurotoxicology. New York, Francis and Taylor, pp 1–35.

Trieberg G (1998) Role of brain imaging techniques in occupational neurotoxicology. In: Costa LG & Manzo L ed. Occupational neurotoxicology. Boca Raton, Florida, CRC Press, pp 199–210.

Tu AT (1995) Neurotoxins from snake venoms. In: Chang LW & Dyer RS ed. Handbook of neurotoxicology. New York, Marcel Dekker, pp 637–665.

US CDC (1991) Preventing lead poisoning in young children. Atlanta, Georgia, US Department of Health and Human Services, Centers for Disease Control.

US EPA (1991a) Pesticide assessment guidelines, subdivision F. Hazard evaluation: Human and domestic animals. Addendum 10: Neurotoxicity, series 81, 82, and 83. Washington, DC, United States Environmental Protection Agency, Office of Prevention, Pesticides and Toxic Substances (EPA No. 540/09-91-123).

US EPA (1991b) Guidelines for developmental toxicity risk assessment. United States Environmental Protection Agency. Fed Regist, **56**: 63798–63826.
US EPA (1991c) Neurotoxicity testing guidelines. United States Environmental Protection Agency. Springfield, Virginia, National Technical Information Service.

US EPA (1995) The use of the benchmark dose approach in health risk assessment. Washington, DC, United States Environmental Protection Agency (EPA/630/R-94-007).

US EPA (1998a) Guidelines for neurotoxicity risk assessment. United States Environmental Protection Agency. Fed Regist, **63**: 26926–26951.

US EPA (1998b) Endocrine Disruptor Screening and Testing Advisory Committee (EDSTAC) final report. Washington, DC, United States Environmental Protection Agency.

US FDA (1970) Guidelines for food additives and contaminants. Rockville, Maryland, United States Food and Drug Administration.

US NRC (1983) Risk assessment in the federal government. Washington, DC, United States National Research Council, National Academy Press.

US NRC (1984) Toxicity testing: Strategies to determine needs and priorities. Washington, DC, United States National Research Council, National Academy of Sciences.

US NRC (1992) Environmental neurotoxicology. Washington, DC, United States National Research Council, National Academy of Sciences, National Academy Press.

US NRC (1993) Pesticides in the diets of infants and children. Washington, DC, United States National Research Council, National Academy of Sciences.

US NRC (1999) Hormonally active agents in the environment. Washington, DC, United States National Research Council, National Academy Press.

US NRC (2000) Scientific frontiers in developmental toxicology and risk assessment. Washington, DC, United States National Research Council, National Academy Press.

US OTA (1990) Neurotoxicity: Identifying and controlling poisons of the nervous system. US Congress, Office of Technology Assessment (OTA-BA-436). Washington, DC, US Government Printing Office.

Valciukas JA (1991) Foundations of environmental and occupational neurotoxicology. New York, Van Nostrand Reinhold.

Van der Laan G, van Dun RECS, Roos Y, Huy T, Wekking EM, Hooisma J, Kulig BM, Emmen HH, Monster AC, & de Wolf FA (1995) [Solvent-induced organic psychosyndrome? A diagnostic protocol.] Den Haag, Ministerie van Sociale Zaken en Werkgelegenheid S-186, Sdu Uitgevers (in Dutch).

Viaene MK, Masschelein R, Leenders J, De Groof M, Swerts LJ, & Roels HA (2000) Neurobehavioural effects of occupational exposure to cadmium: A cross sectional epidemiological study. Occup Environ Med, **57**: 19–27.

Vigliani EC (1954) Carbon disulfide poisoning in viscose rayon factories. Br J Ind Med, **11**: 325–344.

Vorhees CV (1985) Behavioral effects of prenatal d-amphetamine in rats: A parallel trial to the Collaborative Behavioral Teratology Study. Neurobehav Toxicol Teratol, **7**(6): 709–716.

Vorhees CV (1987) Reliability, sensitivity and validity of indices of neurotoxicity. Neurotoxicol Teratol, **9**: 445–464.

Walker CH, Faustman WO, Fowler SC, Kazar DB (1981) A multivariate analysis of some operant variables used in behavioural pharmacology. Psychopharmacology, **74**: 182–186.

Walsh TJ & Tilson HA (1986) The use of pharmacological challenges. In: Annau Z ed. Neurobehavioural toxicology. Baltimore, Maryland, Johns Hopkins Press, pp 244–267.

Walum E, Nordin M, Beckman M, & Odland L (1993) Cellular methods for identification of neurotoxic chemicals and estimation of neurotoxicological risk. Toxicol *In Vitro*, 7: 321–326.

Warren JS (1990) Interleukins and tumor necrosis factor in inflammation. Crit Rev Clin Lab Sci, 28: 37–59.

Webster H deF (1975) Peripheral nerve structure. In: Hubbard JI ed. The peripheral nervous system. New York, Plenum Press, pp 36–54.

Weiss B (1988) Neurobehavioral toxicity as a basis for risk assessment. Trends Pharmacol Sci, 9: 59–62.

Weiss B (1990) Risk assessment: The insidious nature of neurotoxicity and the aging basis. Neurotoxicology, 11: 305–313.

Weiss B (1998) A risk assessment perspective on the neurobehavioral toxicity of endocrine disruptors. Toxicol Ind Health, 14: 341–359.

Weiss B (2000) Vulnerability to pesticide neurotoxicity is a lifetime issue. Neurotoxicology, 21: 67–73.

Weiss B & Clarkson TW (1986) Toxic chemical disasters and the implications of Phopal for technology transfer. Milbank Q, 64: 216–240.

White RF (1995) Clinical neuropsychological investigation of solvent neurotoxicity. In: Chang LW & Dyer RS ed. Handbook of neurotoxicology. New York, Marcel Dekker, pp 355–376.

White RF & Proctor SP (1995) Clinico-neuropsychological assessment methods in behavioural neurotoxicology. In: Chang LW & Slikker W ed. Neurotoxicology: Approaches and methods. New York, Academic Press, pp 711–726.

White RF, Feldman RG, & Proctor SP (1992) Neurobehavioral effects of toxic exposures. In: White RF ed. Clinical syndromes in adult neuropsychology. Amsterdam, Elsevier, pp 1–51.

White RF, Feldman RG, Moss MB, & Proctor SP (1993) Magnetic resonance imaging (MRI), neurobehavioral testing and toxic encephalopathy: Two cases. Environ Res, 61: 117–123.

WHO (1995) Guidelines for good clinical practice for trials on pharmaceutical products. Geneva, World Health Organization (WHO Technical Report Series No. 850).

WHO (2000) Guideline document — Evaluation and use of epidemiological evidence for environmental health risk assessment. Copenhagen, World Health Organization Regional Office for Europe.

Williamson AM (1990) The development of a neurobehavioral test battery for use in hazard evaluations in occupational settings. Neurotoxicol Teratol, 12: 509–514.

Willis WD Jr & Grossman RG (1973) Neurotransmission. In: Medical neurobiology; neuro-anatomical and neurophysiological principles basic to clinical neuroscience. St. Louis, Missouri, C.V. Mosby, 457 pp.

Winneke G (1995) Endpoints of developmental neurotoxicity in environmentally exposed children. Toxicol Lett, **77**: 127–136.

Wirsching RJ, Beninger RJ, & Jhamandas K (1984) Differential effects of scopolamine on working and reference memory of rats in the radial arm maze. Pharmacol Biochem Behav, **20**: 659–662.

Wood RW (1982) Stimulus properties of inhaled substances. In: Mitchell CL ed. New York, Raven Press, pp 199–212.

Woolley DE (1995) Organochlorine insecticides: Neurotoxicity and mechanisms of action. In: Chang LW & Dyer RS ed. Handbook of neurotoxicology. New York, Marcel Dekker, pp 475–510.

Wright CDP, Forshaw PJ, & Ray DE (1988) Classification of the actions of ten pyrethroid insecticides in the rat, using the trigeminal reflex and skeletal muscle as test systems. Pestic Biochem Physiol, **30**: 79–86.

Wyllie TD & Morehouse LC (1978) Mycotoxic fungi, mycotoxins, mycotoxicoses, an encyclopedic handbook. Vols. 1–3. New York, Marcel Dekker.

Xu J, Nolan CC, Lister T, Purcell WM, & Ray DE (1998) Intracellular ATP, a switch in the decision between apoptosis and necrosis. Toxicol Lett, **103**: 139–142.

Yamanouchi N, Okada S, Kodama K, & Sato T (1998) Central nervous system impairment caused by chronic solvent abuse — a review of Japanese studies on the clinical and neuroimaging aspects. Addict Biol, **3**: 15–27.

Yang D, Li C, & He F (1996) Electrophysiological studies in rats of acute dimethoate poisoning. Toxicol Lett, **107**: 249–254.

Yokel RA (1983) Repeated systemic aluminum exposure effects on classical conditioning of the rabbit. Neurobehav Toxicol Teratol, **5**: 41–46.

Yokoyama K, Araki S, Murata K, Nishikitani M, Okumura T, Ishimatsu S, Takasu N, & White RF (1998) Chronic neurobehavioural effects of Tokyo subway sarin poisoning in relation to post-traumatic stress disorder. Arch Environ Health, **53**: 249–256.

Yu ACH, Lee YL, & Eng LF (1993) Astrogliosis in culture I: The model and the effect of antisense oligonucleotides on glial fibrillary acidic protein synthesis. J Neurosci Res, **34**(3): 295–303.

Zavalić M, Mandić Z, Bogadi-Šare, & Plavec D (1998) Quantitative assessment of color vision impairment in workers exposed to toluene. Am J Ind Med, **33**: 297–304.

Zenick H (1983) Use of pharmacological challenge to disclose neurobehavioural deficits. Fed Proc, **42**: 3191–3195.

Zhu QZ, Lindenbaum M, Levavasseur F, Jacomy H, & Julien JP (1998) Disruption of the NF-H gene increases axonal microtubule content and velocity of neurofilament transport: relief of axonopathy resulting from the toxin β,β'-iminodipropionitrile. J Cell Biol, **143**: 183–193.

RESUME ET RECOMMANDATIONS

1. Résumé

Depuis qu'en 1986 a été publié dans la série "Critères d'Hygiène de l'Environnement" le document "Principes et méthodes d'évaluation de la neurotoxicité liée à l'exposition aux produits chimiques," la recherche fondamentale en neurobiologie nous a dotés d'outils sensiblement plus performants pour étudier les effets nocifs des substances chimiques sur le système nerveux. Ces progrès se sont traduits par la parution, au plan national et international, d'un certain nombre de recommandations et de guides relatifs aux tests de neurotoxicité et à l'évaluation des risques (notamment sous l'égide de l'Organisation de coopération et de développement économiques) ainsi que par la publication d'études internationales sur la validation des méthodes d'expérimentation neurocomportementale.

En dépit des progrès accomplis dans l'évaluation du risque neurotoxique, on continue de s'interroger un peu partout dans le monde sur les risques de neurotoxicité liés aux produits chimiques. Ce qui est particulièrement préoccupant, c'est l'absence de données concernant la relation possible entre l'exposition à de faibles concentrations de subtances chimiques présentes dans l'environnement et certains effets sur le développement neurocomportemental des enfants ou certaines maladies neurodégénératives affectant les personnes âgées. Seule une faible proportion des produits chimiques existants a fait l'objet d'une évaluation neurotoxicologique suffisante.

En raison de la complexité du système nerveux, il existe quantité de sites potentiels pour l'action neurotoxique et nombre de séquelles possibles. Il n'y aucun organe qui comporte des fonctions cellulaires aussi diversifiées que celles du système nerveux. Les diverses expressions de la neurotoxicité résultent généralement de la différence de sensibilité entre les diverses sous-populations de cellules qui le constituent. Par ailleurs, l'évaluation de la neuroxicité revêt un caractère particulier en raison du rôle joué, au niveau central, par la barrière hémato-encéphalique et au niveau périphérique, par d'autres structures de ce genre, dans la modulation de l'accès au système nerveux de certaines substances chimiques. En outre, à l'extérieur de la barrière, un certain nombre de cellules spécialisées assument des fonctions neuro-immunoendocriniennes d'intégration qui orchestrent de nombreux processus physiologiques, métaboliques et endocriniens. Ces fonctions d'intégration sont d'une importance fondamentale pour les fonctions cognitives et les fonctions nerveuses supérieures, mais on ne sait guère comment elles peuvent être perturbées par l'exposition à des produits chimiques. Contrairement à ce qui se passe dans d'autres tissus, le remplacement ou la régénération des cellules nerveuses est très limité et c'est cet état de choses qui empêche une récupération complète lorsque l'action neurotoxique a eu pour effet la mort cellulaire.

Lorsqu'on évalue le risque neurotoxique, ilest important, pour l'identification de certaines populations réceptives, notamment les jeunes, les personnes âgées et les sujets ayant une prédisposition génétique à des effets toxiques déterminés, d'en connaître les fondements biologiques. Nombre de facteurs dont dépend la sensibilité à l'action neurotoxique sont les mêmes que ceux à prendre en considération dans l'évaluation de la toxicité vis-à-vis d'autres organes cibles que le système nerveux, car ils concernent des processus métaboliques communs à plusieurs systèmes. Cependant, la complexité et les diverses phases du développement postnatal du système nerveux central qui se succèdent selon une chronologie déterminante, peuvent faire que celui-ci réagisse différemment à certains types d'exposition. De même, le vieillissement entraîne une perte de plasticité et une diminution de la capacité compensatoire du système nerveux qui le rendent potentiellement plus sensible aux agressions neurotoxiques.

Les données relatives aux effets des substances chimiques sur l'Homme font souvent défaut ou du moins n'en rend-t-on pas suffisamment compte. La recherche d'effets neurotoxiques dans le cadre d'études sur des sujets humains reste le moyen le plus direct d'évaluer les risques pour la santé, encore que la présence de facteurs de confusion et l'insuffisance des données rendent la tâche difficile. Il est difficile d'établir le niveau d'exposition des sujets humains et l'état neurologique des populations est d'une extrême diversité. Des progrès importants ont néanmoins été accomplis au cours de la décennie écoulée en ce qui concerne la mise au point de méthodes validées pour la mise en évidence d'effets neurotoxiques chez l'Homme. Les données correspondantes sont tirées de situations impliquant une exposition accidentelle ou professionnelle, de compte-rendus de cas, d'examens cliniques, d'études épidémiologiques et d'études sur le terrain ou en laboratoire. Diverses méthodes ont été améliorées et se sont imposées comme les tests neuropsychologiques normalisés, les batteries de tests assistées par ordinateur, les épreuves neurophysiologiques et biochimiques ou certaines techniques élaborées d'imagerie médicale. Ces méthodes, qui permettent d'étudier les divers points d'aboutissement de l'action neurotoxique, fournissent des données précieuses pour l'évaluation du risque.

Dans la plupart des études neurotoxicologiques, il est encore nécessaire d'avoir recours à des modèles animaux expérimentaux. Désormais, on utillise systématiquement, dans l'expérimentation animale, des méthodes éthologiques, biochimiques, électrophysiologiques et histopathologiques, à côté de batteries d'épreuves fonctionnelles, pour identifier et caractériser les effets neurotoxiques. La normalisation et la validation des batteries de tests utilisées dans l'expérimentation animale ont permis d'améliorer la qualité des données utilisables pour l'évaluation du risque. Un certain nombre d'organismes intergouvernementaux ou nationaux ont élaboré des protocoles expérimentaux, des recommandations pour les différents tests ainsi que des méthodgies pour l'étude de la neurotoxicité chez l'animal adulte ou en cours de développement qui reposent sur l'utilisation de ces diverses techniques. Dans les nouvelles directives concernant les études toxicologiques relatives aux effets aigus ou chroniques figurent désormais un certain nombre de points d'aboutissement au niveau comportemental et histopathologique qui ont expressément pour but d'améliorer l'évaluation des effets sur le système nerveux. Les modèles animaux sont largement utilisés pour étudier les différences de sensibilité des organismes en développement aux agressions chimiques, mais les directives concernant l'étude des effets toxiques sur le développement du système nerveux sont compliquées et les résultats obtenus donnent souvent lieu à des interprétations variées. La plupart des méthodologies applicables aux études neurotoxicologiques sont fondées sur une approche hiérarchique des phénomènes. Quoi qu'il en soit, outre les données issues des protocoles expérimentaux, il faut prendre en compte l'ensemble des sources de données existantes (relations structure-réactivité, recherche sur les mécanismes, etc.) pour disposer d'informations approfondies sur tel ou tel type d'effet neurotoxique.

Comme pour d'autres types de toxicité, l'évaluation du potentiel neurotoxique des substances chimiques chez l'animal de laboratoire doit prendre en compte un certain nombre de facteurs qui sont d'une importance déterminante. Il s'agit en particulier de choisir le modèle animal qui convient, de définir par quelles variables l'exposition sera exprimée et quelle sera la méthodologie expérimentale. Par ailleurs, il faut s'assurer de la validité biologique des points d'aboutissement étudiés, recourir à des mesures dûment validées et veiller au contrôle de qualité. Les conditions expérimentales doivent être fixées compte tenu de la voie et du niveau d'exposition possibles chez l'Homme et il faut prendre également en considération toutes les données disponibles concernant la toxicodynamique et la toxicocinétique de la substance à évaluer.

Dans de nombreux pays, on a mis en place des procédures d'évaluation du risque qui comportent l'analyse des données pertinentes : effets biologiques, niveaux d'exposition ou relations dose-réponse concernant tel ou tel produit chimique, afin d'en évaluer qualitativement et quantitativement les conséquences négatives. Ces procédures sont assez semblables et suivent la démarche habituelle : identification du danger, établissement d'une relation dose-réponse, évaluation de l'exposition et caractérisation du risque. Les principes de cette évaluation du risque évoluent rapidement dans le cas de la neurotoxicité, mais cela se limite en général à l'identification qualitative du danger et, dans une certaine mesure, à la détermination de la relation dose-réponse. L'évaluation de l'exposition et la caractérisation du risque ne sont satisfaisantes que dans quelques cas.

Dans ses principes, l'évaluation du risque imputable aux substances neurotoxiques est généralement analogue à celle d'autres effets non néoplasiques, à cela près que dans le cas du système nerveux, il faut accorder une attention particulière à des questions comme la réversibilité, la compensation et la redondance des fonctions. Il est admis que l'évaluation du risque neurotoxique repose sur la détermination de la dose sans effet nocif observable à laquelle on applique ensuite un coefficient d'incertitude empirique pour fixer la limite d'exposition jugée acceptable. L'évaluation de toutes les données disponibles conditionne la validité de l'évaluation du risque. Il faudra affiner les méthodes et les stratégies d'expérimentation animale à mesure que l'on disposera de données et de technologies nouvelles afin d'améliorer la valeur prédictive des modèles animaux par rapport au risque neurotoxique chez l'Homme.

2. Recommandations

Afin de mettre en oeuvre des stratégies efficaces de contrôle et d'intervention destinées à prévenir les accidents neurotoxiques chez l'Homme, il faut mettre en place une base de données appropriée sur la neurotoxicité potentielle des produits chimiques. Les recommandations ci-après devraient permettre d'améliorer cette base de données :

1. Les programmes de surveillance et l'utilisation de procédures normalisées pour le recueil des données sur l'incidence des intoxications et des réactions indésirables aux agents neurotoxiques chez l'Homme doivent être encouragés ou intensifiés.

2. Il est nécessaire de mieux évaluer l'exposition des individus et des populations aux agents neurotoxiques afin de pouvoir déterminer la relation entre l'exposition et l'effet.

3. Il est nécessaire d'effectuer, à partir d'un certain nombre d'hypothèses, des études épidémiologiques et expérimentales sur l'association possible entre l'exposition aux agents neurotoxiques présents dans l'environnement et les maladies neurodégénératives, eu égard en particulier aux populations sensibles et aux interactions entre génome et environnement.

4. Il conviendrait de repérer les biomarqueurs de l'exposition, de l'effet toxique et de la sensibilité aux agents neurotoxiques puis de les développer et de les valider afin de les utiliser dans les études épidémiologiques sur la neurotoxicité.

5. Un effort de recherche s'impose pour mieux repérer les groupes de population qui pourraient être sensibles aux effets des agents neurotoxiques et caractériser les facteurs responsables de cette sensibilité particulière.

6. Il est nécessaire de disposer de méthodes d'analyse normalisées et d'établir des normes pour l'évaluation de la neurotoxicité chez les

nourrissons et les enfants en vue de les utiliser dans des études transculturelles relatives à l'action des agents neurotoxiques sur le système nerveux humain en développement.

7. Il faut faire une plus grande place aux études relatives à l'exposition à des substances ou à des mélanges de substances chimiques lors de la période périnatale afin de définir la sensibilité relative du système nerveux en développement vis-à-vis des agressions neurotoxiques.

8. Il convient de mettre au point des méthodes efficaces d'expérimentation animale et de les valider dans le cadre d'études collectives internationales.

9. Pour établir la signification biologique des modifications subtiles constatées au niveau d'un grand nombre des points d'aboutissement de l'action toxique qui font l'objet d'études neurotoxicologiques, il faut disposer de meilleurs modèles animaux à partir desquels on puisse définir la relation entre les événements survenant au niveau moléculaire ou cellulaire et les manifestations cliniques de la neurotoxicité.

10. Il convient d'encourager les recherches visant à déterminer de quelle manière les substances chimiques peuvent affecter les fonctions intégrées du système nerveux et en particulier, les recherches relatives aux substances qui perturbent le système endocrine.

11. L'utilisation des relations structure-activité pourrait être utile pour déterminer le potentiel neurotoxique d'une substance chimique et c'est un aspect qui est à approfondir.

12. Il existe un certain nombre d'aléas dans le mode d'évaluation actuel du risque neurotoxique, qui tiennent à certaines hypothèses formulées par défaut et aux facteurs ou coefficients d'incertitude utilisés pour l'extrapolation de l'animal à l'Homme et de l'aigu au chronique ou encore pour prendre en compte les variations au sein des population : il importe, pour les réduire, d'entreprendre des recherche dans le but : 1) d'élucider le mécanisme de la neurotoxicité et d'encourager l'utilisation des données mécanistiques dans l'évaluation du risque; 2) d'élaborer des modèles dose-

réponse de nature mécanistique ou des modèles toxicocinétiques permettant l'extrapolation d'une dose, d'une voie d'administration ou d'une espèce à une autre; 3) de moins recourir aux facteurs ou coefficients d'incertitude dans la quantification du risque; 4) de mettre à disposition des procédures d'évaluation du risque améliorées et normalisées et d'en encourager l'usage.

13. Les directives actuelles en matière d'évaluation du risque sont axées sur l'étude d'un seul produit et d'une seule voie d'exposition à la fois. Afin de prendre en compte l'exposition simultanée à plusieurs substances et d'aborder les problèmes de toxicité cumulative, il est nécessaire d'entreprendre des recherches en vue : 1) de vérifier s'il y a effectivement additivité de l'action toxique des substances dont l'action est similaire; 2) d'étudier la possibilité d'interactions non additives éventuelles entre substances chimique ayant des modes d'action différents; 3) d'étudier les interactions potentielles entre plusieurs substances chimiques à des doses inférieures à celles qui sont nécessaires pour produire un effet décelable après une exposition unique.

RESUMEN Y RECOMENDACIONES

1. Resumen

Desde la publicación en 1986 del documento de la serie Criterios de Salud Ambiental del IPCS titulado «Principles and Methods for the Assessment of Neurotoxicity Associated with Exposure to Chemicals», la investigación fundamental en neurobiología ha mejorado notablemente nuestra capacidad para evaluar los efectos perjudiciales de las sustancias químicas sobre el sistema nervioso. Este progreso se refleja en la existencia de varias directrices nacionales e internacionales (p. ej., de la Organización de Cooperación y Desarrollo Económicos) relativas a los ensayos de neurotoxicidad, así como pautas y orientaciones para la evaluación del riesgo, y estudios internacionales de validación de los tests neurocomportamentales.

Pese a los progresos logrados en la evaluación del riesgo de neurotoxicidad, persiste en todo el mundo la inquietud por los posibles efectos neurotóxicos de las sustancias químicas. Preocupa especialmente la ausencia de datos sobre las presuntas relaciones entre la exposición a concentraciones bajas de sustancias químicas medioambientales y su repercusión tanto en el desarrollo neurocomportamental del niño como en las enfermedades neurodegenerativas del anciano. Sólo se ha evaluado satisfactoriamente la neurotoxicidad de un pequeño número de sustancias químicas.

La complejidad del sistema nervioso determina la existencia de numerosos blancos potenciales y secuelas. Ningún otro sistema orgánico posee tan amplia variedad de funciones celulares especializadas. Las distintas expresiones de la neurotoxicidad se deben generalmente a las distintas sensibilidades de las diversas subpoblaciones de células que constituyen el sistema nervioso. El estado y la función de la barrera hematoencefálica del sistema nervioso central (SNC), y de estructuras similares del sistema nervioso periférico, en la modulación del acceso de algunas sustancias químicas al sistema nervioso son también cuestiones específicas que deben tenerse en cuenta al evaluar la neurotoxicidad. Además, algunas células especializadas situadas fuera de la barrera ejercen importantes funciones de integración neuroinmunoendocrina que coordinan numerosos procesos fisiológicos, metabólicos y endocrinos. Estas intervenciones integradoras son fundamentales para la cognición y otras funciones neurales de orden superior, pero los conocimientos acerca de cómo pueden verse alteradas por la exposición a sustancias químicas son limitados. A diferencia de lo que ocurre en otros tejidos, la capacidad de las neuronas para sustituir a las dañadas o regenerarse es muy restringida, y constituye un factor limitante para conseguir la plena recuperación tras una agresión neurotóxica causante de muerte celular.

El fundamento biológico para la identificación de ciertas poblaciones sensibles, como los jóvenes, los ancianos y las personas predispuestas genéticamente a ciertas formas de toxicidad, es un aspecto importante de la evaluación del riesgo neurotóxico. Muchos de los factores que confieren sensibilidad a la neurotoxicidad no diferirán de los que deben tenerse en consideración al evaluar el riesgo de toxicidad para otros órganos diana, ya que intervienen procesos metabólicos comunes a muchos sistemas orgánicos. Sin embargo, es muy probable que, debido a la complejidad del largo proceso de desarrollo postnatal del SNC y a la decisiva importancia de la puntual sucesión de sus acontecimientos, el sistema nervioso en desarrollo sea especialmente sensible a ciertas exposiciones. Del mismo modo, al reducir la plasticidad y la capacidad compensadora del sistema nervioso, el envejecimiento incrementa la potencial sensibilidad de éste a las agresiones neurotóxicas.

Es frecuente que los datos sobre los efectos de las sustancias químicas en los seres humanos no estén disponibles, o bien informen de un número de casos inferior al real. La detección de la neurotoxicidad en estudios en seres humanos constituye el medio más directo de evaluar los riesgos para la salud, pero se complica a menudo por factores de confusión y datos insuficientes. Es difícil determinar los niveles de exposición en los seres humanos, y el estado neurológico de las poblaciones es sumamente heterogéneo. Sin embargo, en el último decenio se han logrado importantes avances en la puesta a punto de métodos validados para detectar la neurotoxicidad en seres humanos. Los datos proceden de exposiciones accidentales y laborales, estudios de casos, evaluaciones clínicas, estudios epidemiológicos, y estudios de laboratorio y sobre el terreno. Se ha mejorado y confirmado la eficacia de tests neuropsicológicos normalizados, de baterías de pruebas informatizadas y validadas, y de determinaciones neurofisiológicas y bioquímicas, así como de técnicas refinadas de diagnóstico por la imagen. Estos métodos pueden utilizarse en la evaluación de diversas variables de la neurotoxicidad humana y han aportado datos útiles para determinar el riesgo neurotóxico.

La mayoría de las evaluaciones neurotoxicológicas siguen dependiendo de la información proporcionada por los modelos animales. Hoy día, en los estudios con animales se aplican sistemáticamente métodos comportamentales, bioquímicos, electrofisiológicos e histopatológicos, así como baterías de pruebas funcionales validadas, para identificar y caracterizar los efectos neurotóxicos. La normalización y la validación de las baterías de pruebas en animales han mejorado la calidad de los datos disponibles para la evaluación del riesgo. Tanto organizaciones intergubernamentales como gobiernos nacionales han combinado de diversas maneras estos métodos con objeto de formular protocolos, directrices y estrategias específicos y orientados a determinar la neurotoxicidad en animales adultos y en desarrollo. En la actualidad, las nuevas directrices para los estudios normalizados de toxicidad aguda y de dosis repetidas comprenden también variables comportamentales e histopatológicas cuya finalidad específica es perfeccionar la evaluación de sistema nervioso. Aunque se han utilizado mucho los modelos animales para estudiar la sensibilidad diferencial de los organismos en desarrollo a las agresiones de sustancias químicas, las directrices actuales para el estudio de la neurotoxicidad durante el desarrollo son complejas, y a menudo los resultados son objeto de interpretaciones diversas. La mayor parte de las estrategias de determinación de la neurotoxicidad se basan en un esquema jerárquico o escalonado. Sin embargo, para obtener información exhaustiva sobre un tipo concreto de efecto neurotóxico, además de los datos de los protocolos de pruebas, deben tenerse en cuenta todas las fuentes de datos disponibles (relaciones estructura–actividad, investigaciones sobre mecanismos de acción, etc.).

Al igual que ocurre en otras toxicidades, existen diversos factores de crucial importancia para evaluar el potencial neurotóxico de sustancias químicas en animales de experimentación, a saber: la correcta selección de los modelos animales, las variables relativas a la exposición y los métodos de prueba, un acuerdo sobre la pertinencia biológica de las variables elegidas, el empleo de medidas validadas y la garantía de la calidad. Las condiciones experimentales deben tener en cuenta las posibles vías y concentraciones de la exposición humana, así como toda la información toxicodinámica y toxicocinética disponible.

Muchos países han elaborado procesos de evaluación del riesgo en los que se analizan los datos relativos a los efectos biológicos de una sustancia química concreta, a las relaciones dosis–respuesta y a la exposición, a fin de establecer estimaciones cualitativas y cuantitativas de los resultados adversos. Estos procesos son bastante similares y consisten por lo general en identificar los riesgos, evaluar la relación entre dosis y respuesta, y determinar el riesgo. Aunque, en el terreno concreto de la neurotoxicidad, los principios de la evaluación del riesgo están evolucionando rápidamente, todavía se limitan por lo general a la identificación cualitativa del riesgo y, en cierta medida, a la determinación de la relación dosis–respuesta. Sólo unos pocos procesos abordan satisfactoriamente la evaluación de la exposición o la caracterización del riesgo.

La aplicación de los principios de evaluación del riesgo para sustancias químicas neurotóxicas es similar a la de otras variables de carácter no canceroso, con la salvedad de que debe prestarse especial atención a aspectos del sistema nervioso tales como la reversibilidad, la compensación y la redundancia de funciones. Las evaluaciones del riesgo neurotoxicológico se han basado convencionalmente en las concentraciones a las que no se observan efectos adversos, así como en factores empíricos de incertidumbre, para derivar límites de exposición aceptables. La clave de unas evaluaciones del riesgo bien fundadas reside en considerar todos los datos disponibles. Deben perfeccionarse constantemente los métodos y estrategias de prueba en animales de laboratorio a medida que se dispone de nuevos datos y tecnologías, para mejorar la validez predictiva de los modelos animales en la evaluación del riesgo de neurotoxicidad humana.

2. Recomendaciones

La aplicación de estrategias eficaces de control e intervención para la prevención de la neurotoxicidad humana requiere poner a punto una base de conocimientos suficiente sobre la potencial neurotoxicidad de las sustancias químicas. Con el propósito de mejorar esta base de conocimientos, se formulan las recomendaciones siguientes:

1. Deberían promoverse y fortalecerse los programas de vigilancia, así como el uso de formatos armonizados para la recogida de datos sobre la incidencia de intoxicaciones y de reacciones adversas a sustancias neurotóxicas en seres humanos.

2. Se precisa una mejor evaluación de la exposición de los individuos y las poblaciones a las sustancias neurotóxicas, a fin de analizar las relaciones entre exposición y efecto.

3. Se precisan estudios epidemiológicos y experimentales basados en hipótesis sobre el posible nexo entre exposiciones medioambientales y enfermedades neurodegenerativas, especialmente en lo relativo a las poblaciones sensibles y las interacciones entre los genes y el medio ambiente.

4. Se deberían identificar, desarrollar y validar biomarcadores de exposición, de efecto y de sensibilidad, para su utilización en estudios epidemiológicos de neurotoxicidad.

5. Se precisan investigaciones para identificar mejor las subpoblaciones potencialmente sensibles a los efectos de sustancias neurotóxicas, así como para caracterizar los factores que contribuyen a incrementar la sensibilidad.

6. Se precisan pruebas normalizadas, así como normas de evaluación de la neurotoxicidad en lactantes y niños, con objeto de aplicarlas a estudios transculturales sobre neurotoxicidad en el desarrollo humano.

7. Debe prestarse mayor atención a los estudios sobre la exposición perinatal a sustancias químicas o a mezclas de ellas, para definir la sensibilidad relativa del sistema nervioso en desarrollo a la agresión neurotóxica.

8. Es necesario concebir pruebas eficientes en animales para estudiar la neurotoxicidad durante el desarrollo, y validarlas en estudios internacionales en colaboración.

9. Para determinar la importancia biológica de las ligeras modificaciones que experimentan muchas de las variables utilizadas en las

investigaciones neurotoxicológicas se necesitan mejores modelos animales, que ayuden a determinar las relaciones entre los fenómenos moleculares/celulares y las manifestaciones clínicas de la neurotoxicidad.

10. Debería promoverse la investigación del efecto de las sustancias químicas sobre las funciones integradas del sistema nervioso, en particular los estudios sobre los perturbadores endocrinos.

11. Es preciso examinar más detenidamente el interés de aplicar las relaciones entre estructura y actividad a la determinación del potencial neurotóxico de las sustancias químicas.

12. Es preciso reducir las incertidumbres de la actual evaluación del riesgo de neurotoxicidad, debidas a que ésta depende de presunciones por defecto y de factores de incertidumbre para extrapolar de los animales a los seres humanos y de la exposición aguda a la crónica, así como explicar la variabilidad intrapoblacional. Son necesarias, pues, investigaciones para (1) definir los mecanismos de neurotoxicidad y promover el uso de datos explicativos en la evaluación del riesgo; (2) proporcionar modelos de la relación dosis–respuesta basados en los mecanismos de acción y modelos toxicocinéticos que permitan extrapolar la dosis, la vía y la especie; (3) reducir el empleo de factores de incertidumbre en las estimaciones cuantitativas del riesgo; y (4) promover la disponibilidad y el uso de procedimientos de evaluación del riesgo perfeccionados y armonizados.

13. Las actuales directrices de evaluación del riesgo se centran en evaluar una única sustancia química tras la exposición por una vía también única. El problema de la exposición combinada o de la toxicidad acumulada exige llevar a cabo investigaciones para (1) probar la hipótesis de la aditividad de las sustancias químicas que comparten un modo de acción similar; (2) evaluar las posibles interacciones no aditivas de las sustancias químicas con modos de acción distintos; y (3) estudiar las interacciones potenciales de varias sustancias químicas en dosis inferiores a las necesarias para que cada una de ellas por separado produzca efectos detectables.